Anaesthesia OSCE 2nd Edition

Dedication

To Menai, Gareth, Ceri, Owen and Bethan.
To Mohamed, Naeima, Taha, Liyean and Hala.

We do not teach we only help you to learn.

Anaesthesia OSCE
2nd Edition

G Arthurs FRCA
Consultant Anaesthetist
Maelor Hospital
Wrexham

K M Elfituri FRCA FFARCSI
Associate Specialist
Maelor Hospital
Wrexham

Illustrations by
T Bailey RGN RNM Cert Ed
Maelor Hospital
Wrexham

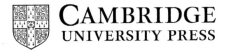
CAMBRIDGE
UNIVERSITY PRESS

CAMBRIDGE UNIVERSITY PRESS
Cambridge, New York, Melbourne, Madrid, Cape Town, Singapore, São Paulo

Cambridge University Press
The Edinburgh Building, Cambridge CB2 2RU, UK

Published in the United States of America by Cambridge University Press, New York

www.cambridge.org
Information on this title: www.cambridge.org/9780521681827

© Greenwich Medical Media Ltd 2002

The rights of G Arthurs and K Elfituri to be identified as authors of this work have been asserted
by them in accordance with the Copyright, Designs and Patents Act 1988.

First published 2002
Reprinted 2004
Digitally reprinted by Cambridge University Press 2006

A catalogue record for this publication is available from the British Library

ISBN-13 978-0-521-68182-7 paperback
ISBN-10 0-521-68182-0 paperback

CONTENTS

13. ECG

14. Data

PREFACE

The second edition of The Anaesthesia OSCE has been revised and greatly expanded to include new material. The aim is, as in the original, to act as an aid for those sitting this new type of examination and to help trainers to prepare practice OSCE stations.

There has been an increase in the number of stations to 16. The OSCE Examination tests a variety of abilities which are reflected in the different stations. Some sections are of a conventional nature with questions on data, ECGs or CXRs. Other stations involve role play and explanations. The introduction to each section has been developed to give more guidance on the relevant knowledge and approach to be used.

Some of the scenarios have been posed as a question and then a tutorial. It is suggested that whenever possible, candidates practice with a friend playing the part of the patient as illustrated in the text. No two patients are the same so dealing with various interpretations of a scene will help fine tune the responses.

Teaching and learning should be enjoyable. A number of quizzes have been retained to highlight the defects in apparatus. This is to help trainees to get used to testing apparatus or to assemble it correctly.

Many trainers are still unfamiliar with the OSCE style of examination. The information is presented in short bites which are suitable for a 5–10 minute tutorial. They can also be added together to enable a trainer to make up a mock examination.

ACKNOWLEDGEMENTS

We acknowledge and thank all those who have made this book possible. The co-authors of the first edition K Eggers and J Everatt; Gavin Smith and Gill Clark of GMM; Debra Barrie, freelance copy-editor; Nora Naughton of Naughton Project Management and the support we have received from our anaesthetic colleagues and families.

INTRODUCTION

The objective structured clinical examination (OSCE) has been introduced into postgraduate examinations for a number of reasons. It is a way of examining skills such as communication, attitude, clinical tasks and history taking in a way that were not examined in the past. The marking is predetermined and objective. Unless a candidate deals with a particular aspect of the problem, they do not score that point. This reduces examiner bias and leads to a fairer examination.

The purpose of this book is to help candidates preparing for an OSCE examination to understand the type of station they might encounter. It also aims to help tutors to set a trial examination. Practise of any skill leads to perfection. Practise of a wrong technique or skill not only leads to poor medical practice but also to failure in the examination.

An anaesthetist is a doctor first and then an anaesthetist. When doctors fail it is as much in their ability to say what they are doing as in the doing of a practical task. An ability to find out what a patient is anxious about and to explain the problem in simple language is as important in clinical practice as being able to perform a complicated technical task.

A system is essential and it is vital that the system has been practised to the point that it becomes automatic. Systems can be applied to resuscitation, history taking, measuring the blood pressure and checking the anaesthetic machine to name just a few tasks. Without a system, a doctor will jump at different points with the end result of missing points and taking longer to cover the same ground. Time is short in real life and in the examination.

Lack of practice is a sure way to fail an examination. Most experience will be gained in everyday tasks but these and less often performed tasks will be improved by mock examinations and the presence of an observer to comment on performance.

Stations that require explanation to a patient can be rehearsed with a tutor to ensure that your system is working.

The logistics of the examination

The OSCE is made up of a number of stations. The guidance of the *Royal College of Anaesthetists Examinations Regulations* should be read for the latest details. Past regulations indicate that there will be 16 stations, each one lasting 5 minutes with a 90-second break between each station. There are rest stations. You may become quite dry with talking so drinking water is available at the rest stations. In the 90-second break try to put the last station out of your mind and read the instructions for the next station. Consider how you will approach the next problem and what issues are involved. Each station is marked independently of the other stations. It is necessary to pass most of the stations in order to pass the examination but do not give up if one station goes badly. All stations carry equal importance. Some stations may include negative marking but if they do not then it is worth a guess. Check carefully if there is negative marking at any station.

It is probably best to dress tidily but in clothing that is suitable for moving around and for demonstrating resuscitation of a manikin that will probably be on the floor. Do not carry heavy bags or coats from one station to the next, leave them in the cloakroom provided. Take only your identification label, a biro and stethoscope in a pocket.

At the beginning every candidate is taken into a waiting booth. Read the instructions about this station at which you are going to start. Some candidates will start in a rest station. When the bell rings or whistle sounds you move to the station and the examination starts.

The role of an examiner varies between stations. Some stations are like an MCQ with data presented for you to read and then a series of questions. At other stations you will be asked to perform a task and an examiner will observe your actions. At another station, an examiner may ask questions about a topic.

The types of station you will encounter are:

History taking

Take a comprehensive but relevant history. Relevant to the current situation means: identify the main and any secondary condition(s). What is the current complaint and are there any related problems?

History taking should start with the present condition. Ask, "What is your main complaint?" or, "Why are you in hospital?" If the problem is less obvious ask, "What are you worried about?" and wait for an answer. Let the patient explain their problem. If the person is wandering away from the point bring them back to the main issue. After the main issue has been explored ask if there are any supplementary or allied issues. The cataract patient may be diabetic; the vascular patient is likely to have arteriosclerosis in all vessels.

Then ask about the past history, including anaesthetics. Systematically ask about symptoms from the various organs and systems of the body, drugs and allergies and social history including alcohol, smoking, other drugs and possible risk of hepatitis. Do not forget to ask about anaesthetic-related items such as teeth, veins, postoperative nausea and vomiting. By the end of the history you should have a differential diagnosis of what is wrong.

You may not like the idea of role-play but by pretending to be the patient for a friend while they test their skills, and then they in turn for you, will give you insight into the problem.

Physical examination

There will be a patient for you to examine. It is vital to be able to demonstrate a correct and logical technique. You may be asked to examine a whole system such as the respiratory system or part of a system such as the pulse, the blood pressure or the heart. The nervous system may be divided into the cranial nerves and the peripheral nervous system.

Communication skills

The skills being tested are your ability to listen carefully to patients and to identify their problem(s). A number of approaches may be relevant. Do not impose your ideas on the patient. You may need to give a comprehensive explanation, check that the patient understands and leave time for any extra worries the patient may have. The patient may express strong emotion such as anxiety, worry or anger. Try to find out why they feel the way they do and respond appropriately with reassurance, sympathy for their situation or comfort. Then go on to say how the situation will be resolved. You are being tested on your attitude and the way you deal with a patient and also the content of what you are saying. While it is important to listen, it is also important to give accurate, adequate and understandable explanations. Check: Have I listened to the patient's problem? Have I understood what they are concerned about? Have I offered the correct advice or information?

Do not be frightened to suggest that you will seek more information or you will come back later to check everything is understood.

Resuscitation

You will be asked to demonstrate a resuscitation technique you will use for a collapsed child, adult or mother using a manikin. You may be asked to complete one of the algorithms for managing a cardiac dysrhythmia. The recommendations of the Resuscitation Council should be followed exactly.

Anaesthetic apparatus

The apparatus may need setting up or testing. There may be pictures of apparatus with a series of questions or actual equipment such as an anaesthetic machine, breathing circuit or tracheal tube. Use the Association of Anaesthetists checklist for the anaesthetic machine to the letter. There may be a missing Bodok seal or ring from the selectatec fitting. Know about soda lime and circle systems. Practice and understand each piece of equipment, how it works, how to test it is safe to use and what may go wrong. It is likely that you are used to an ODA or nurse who prepares the equipment for you. Pretend you are the ODA and do it yourself. Find out how everything works and is checked or set up.

Monitoring and measuring apparatus

Anaesthetists have available to them a wide range of apparatus to measure many different physiological parameters. Know how each works, the physical principles, and the problems with their use in clinical practice.

Anaesthetic hazards

Know about the use and problems of electrical apparatus such as diathermy and defibrillation. It is not enough just to turn them on. Know how they work, how to use them safely and any problems with their use.

Skill station

This is a hands on demonstration of a skill on a manikin, such as cricothyroid puncture or any local anaesthetic technique from the head to the ankle. Plenty of anatomical background may come in here.

Statistics

You are expected to have a basic understanding of statistical principles: the methodology behind setting up and conducting a clinical trial; the way in which data is classified and the tests that can be used to assess significance. A test of statistical analysis may be presented as the results of a trial.

Data interpretation

There may be an ECG, X-ray of chest, skull or spine, results from haematology, biochemistry, arterial blood gases, and pulmonary or cardiac function. Be prepared to recognise CT or MRI scans of the head, thorax or abdomen, a coronary angiogram or echo examination of the heart. Check for negative marking and, if none exists, guess.

HISTORY TAKING

1

Introduction

There is a finite amount of time in which to obtain all the facts that you require. In the OSCE this is 5 minutes. Limit yourself to taking a history, do not start to examine the pulse, or explain a symptom as part of history taking. The examiner will check your examination number before you start. While you are waiting to see the patient, plan your questions in relation to the scenario you are given. Think about the case and the questions that are relevant to this condition as well as the general screening questions. One example is the diabetic patient who may have vascular, eye, renal and neurological disorders, but may present as a cataract patient and you forget to ask whether the patient is diabetic.

Allow the patient time to tell their story. Do not cut across the story too early, you may miss a vital piece of information. As the story unfolds, think of further questions or side issues. Try to ask open-ended questions. These are questions that cannot be answered by "Yes" or "No". For instance: "Tell me about your condition?" "How does the pain affect you?" "What other operations have you had?" "Why were/are you in hospital?" "How long have you been in hospital and what have they been doing to you?" "What have they told you is wrong?" Not: "Did you have an operation in the past? Answer: "Yes" or "No".

General approach to patient
- Greet the patient appropriately, e.g. "Good morning".
- Introduce yourself by name, the patient should know who is their doctor.
- Be confident but quietly friendly.
- Make sure the patient is comfortable.
- If appropriate, shake the patient's hand but do not waste time.

Take a relevant history. Have an order for your questioning, e.g.:

- Present complaint
- History of present illness
- Systematic review
- Past medical history
- Family history
- Personal and social history
- Drugs and medicines

■ Allergies
■ Specific anaesthetic points.

Present complaint
Find out what is the principle symptom by asking:

■ What is your main complaint?
■ What operation are you going to have? Which side is it?
■ Why are you seeing a doctor?

History of present illness
Determine the chronology of the illness by asking:

■ How and when did your illness or symptoms start?
■ When did you first notice anything wrong?
■ When were you last perfectly well?

With each symptom determine:

■ Duration
■ Onset – Sudden or gradual
■ Relieving or aggravating factors
■ Spread or radiation.

What has happened since the first time?

■ Constant, variable, periodic
■ Frequency
■ Getting worse or better
■ Relieving or aggravating factors
■ Associated symptoms
■ Treatments received.

Systematic review
Whenever a positive answer is given, always follow this up by obtaining more relevant details.

General questions
Ask about the following:

■ Appetite: Is it normal, increased or reduced?
■ Weight: What is it? Is your weight steady, increasing or are you losing weight?
■ General well-being: Do you feel ill or well, weak or tired?
■ Sleep: Is sleep disturbed by night sweats (could be TB or other chronic infection, or a haematological condition), pain or nocturia, snoring (possible difficult intubation and CVS strain)?
■ Aches and pains.

The order in which you ask about different systems may be determined by the initial symptoms.

Cardiovascular system

Ask about:

- Chest pain: Is it central or left chest with radiation to neck or arm, related to exercise, relieved by rest?
- Cough, either dry or frothy and blood-stained with pulmonary oedema.
- Exercise tolerance:
  - How many stairs can you climb before stopping? (Normal people can climb one flight on their oxygen reserve. It is only the second flight that normally causes breathlessness.)
  - How far can you walk on the flat?
- Short of breath or breathlessness:
  - When? At rest or on exercise?
  - Breathless on lying flat – orthopnoea
  - Breathless at night – paroxysmal nocturnal dyspnoea (PND)
- Do you have breathlessness in bed? What do you do? (PND patients get out and stand by an open window.)
- How many pillows do you use in bed?
- Palpitations: Are you aware of your heart beating?
- Ankle swelling: Do your ankles swell? One or both? (May be due to RVF, poor lymphatic or venous drainage.)
- Black outs or dizzy spells: Differentiate among
  - faint – possible blood loss
  - anaemia – recover quickly
  - low cardiac output – tired and weak all day
  - carotid or vertebral stenosis – symptoms when looking up at ceiling
  - epilepsy
  - diabetes.
  - Have you had black outs? What happens? Are you describing what you remember or what others tell you happens?

Respiratory symptoms

- Cough: Dry or productive of sputum. If productive, which time of day is it most? What is the colour? How much?
  - Productive cough – bronchitis = a productive cough for more than 3 months in a year, for more than 2 years in succession. Often flecked with blood.
  - Colour: Infected; yellow or green. Is there underlying bronchiectasis?
- Blood in sputum. Amount can differentiate between bronchitis and heart failure with flecked sputum or more with carcinoma or tuberculosis.
- Dyspnoea: respiratory cause if not affected by lying down, but by exercise.
- Wheeze: inspiratory upper airway; expiratory lower airways

Central nervous system

Ask about the following:

- Headaches: Do you have headaches? If so where are they, constant or variable, nature, time of day? Early morning with vomiting suggests raised intracranial pressure.

- Fits (differentiated from faints.): Have you had any blackouts, unexplained loss of consciousness? Epilepsy occurs in 1 : 200 but has implications for employment so some people may be reluctant to admit to fits.
- Dizziness: Abnormal sensations sitting or standing? These could be related to ear problems.
- Unsteady gait: Do you have difficulty walking due to steadiness as opposed to arthritis? In the elderly, think of CVA, Parkinsonism; in all ages, intracranial lesions.
- Sleep: Do you sleep normally or are you awake? If awake, is it due to a symptom?

Gastro intestinal tract
- Indigestion: Do you suffer from heartburn or water brash? Abdominal pain related to eating? Is there a risk of regurgitation?
- Nausea and vomiting: Do you feel, or are you sick? (This can occur with gastritis, intestinal obstruction, hypercalcaemia or other electrolyte abnormality, raised intracranial pressure, pregnancy.)
- Bowel habit: Constipation or diarrhoea?
- Jaundice: Have you been jaundiced (yellow)? Are your stools pale, urine pale and floating?

Genito-urinary
- Nocturia is a symptom of poor renal concentrating capacity. If present it implies reduced renal function, high fluid intake or diabetes.
- Colour of urine: Concentrated, blood, porphyrins, infection.
- Pain in loin or back: From the kidney or stones.
- Menstruation: Periods regular and the amount of blood loss.

Musculo-skeletal
Do you have:
- Painful joints?
- Stiffness or swelling?
- Limited neck and jaw movement or mouth opening?

Past medical history
- Have you had any serious illness in the past?
- Have you had any operations and anaesthetics? If so what were they, were there any complications?
- Were there any problems?
- Do you suffer from?
  - Diabetes
  - Hypertension
  - Chest / heart problems
  - Epilepsy.

Family history
- Are there any illnesses that run in your family?

- Have any family members had operations/anaesthetic and were there any problems? Exclude suxamethonium apnoea and malignant hypertension.
- Are your parents still alive? What did they die of?

Personal and social history
- Smoking: How many of what and for how long? Is there a possibility of related diseases, bronchitis, Ca lung, and arteriosclerosis?
- Alcohol intake: How much, what and how often? Associated problems or liver impairment, gastritis, oesophageal varices.
- Possibility of AIDS or hepatitis.
  - Does your social life lead you to be at risk from AIDS or hepatitis?
  - Do you use recreational drugs?

Drugs and medicines
- Please tell me about all the drugs and medicines you are taking?
- Have you had any side-effects to a drug?
- Have there been any recent changes in prescribing, if yes, why?
- Remember to ask about the contraceptive pill and HRT.
- Does the patient carry an alert card or badge?

Allergies
- Are you allergic to anything, including drugs?
- How did this present or affect you? Did you collapse or have a rash?

Specific anaesthetic points
- Difficult teeth
- Regurgitation
- Airway neck movement, mouth opening, snoring.
- Past nausea and vomiting
- Venous access
- Risk of DVT.

A Child
Different information is required from a parent about a child. A child may be a poor historian and will not usually have the same symptoms as an adult. They are more likely to have a congenital condition and less likely to have a past medical history.

The birth
- Were there any difficulties in the pregnancy or at the delivery/birth?
- Were any abnormalities found at birth? (This is the time that congenital problems will be identified.)
- Has the child been growing and developing normally? (Failure to attain milestones and failure to thrive are non-specific indicators that something is wrong.)
- Are there any loose teeth? What will venous access be like?

Points to remember

In real life we like a patient to have one condition. In an examination a patient can have a second, possibly unrelated problem, or a twist to the history.

Think of relationships. If there have been previous operations: what were they, were there any problems? Gastrectomy may be followed by anaemia due to diet or megaloblastic changes related to loss of intrinsic factor. Thyroidectomy patients may have an increased or reduced thyroid function as well as a recurrent nerve lesion from surgery. Hernia patients may have an associated intra-abdominal tumour. Patients with rheumatoid arthritis or diabetes may have problems with many systems.

Smokers may have lung cancer and smoking is linked to drinking alcohol, which may lead to oesophageal varices or liver disease. There is a relationship between smoking, taking recreational drugs of addiction and a high alcohol intake. Do not forget to ask about alcohol intake. After alcohol think of recreational drugs, exposure to hepatitis and possible AIDS infection. These conditions are no respecter of social class, anyone can be affected. If in doubt ask: "Do you use drugs other than for your health?" or, "Are you at risk from having AIDS or hepatitis (have you been yellow or had jaundice)?"

Certain jobs are associated with diseases such as asbestosis and mesothelioma, cancer of the bladder and working with dyes, dust diseases of the lung from mining, allergic alveolitis from farmers' lung and birds like pigeons.

Examples of history taking

Case 1: A relevant history from a patient who has had a myocardial infarction (MI)

1. Pain
   - Onset: rest or exercise
   - Location
   - Duration usually over half an hour, less if angina
   - Quality, crushing, compressing
   - Exacerbation, increased with work
   - Alleviation, angina GTN
   - Radiation, neck and arm
   - Quantity, can be mild to severe.

Associated symptoms
2. Breathlessness. About one-quarter of all cases describe an acute attack of dyspnoea as a feature of the attack
3. Cold sweat often associated with nausea and vomiting
4. Pallor, normally reported by witnesses
5. Previous attacks of angina
6. Past medical history
   - Hypertensive
   - Stroke
   - Diabetes mellitus
   - Contraceptive pills
   - Symptoms of paroxysmal nocturnal dyspnoea
   - Snoring and sleep apnoea
7. Family history
   - Myocardial infarction
   - Diabetes mellitus
   - Hypertension
   - Raised cholesterol
   - Gout
8. Other risk factors
   - Smoking
   - Stress/occupation
9. If the MI was a while ago: If 3–6 months have passed it should not be assumed that an operation is safe. Are there any complications? What is the exercise tolerance? Is there evidence of heart failure, rupture valve cusps, ventricular failure/aneurysm, embolic phenomena or dysrhythmias?

Case 2: A patient who has a pacemaker

1. Why was the pacemaker fitted?
2. Is the patient pacemaker-dependent?
3. Has the pacemaker been checked during the last year and found to operate without problems?

4. Does the patient have associated heart disease (IHD/CHF)?
5. Does the patient experience any symptoms, which might be due to pacemaker malfunction?
   - Syncope
   - Dizziness
   - Palpitation
   - Angina.

All pacemaker patients are given an European pacemaker identification card, which contains information about

- Make of pacemaker
- Pacemaker leads (uni/bipolar)
- Date and place of implant
- Implanting cardiologist
- Pacing mode
- Pacing rate
- Reason for pacemaker implant and symptomatology
- Follow-up data.

Case 3: A patient with asthma
1. How did it start?
2. When did it start?
3. Frequency and severity of attacks
4. Factors provoking attacks
   - Upper respiratory tract infection
   - Seasonal (allergic to pollen)
   - Cold
   - Exercise
   - Food
   - House dust
   - Emotion
   - Drugs
   - Smoke
   - Drugs NSAIDs
5. Past medical history. Has there been a need for hospitalisation and ventilation.
6. Drug history
   - Bronchodilator therapy
   - Steroids
7. Family history
   - Asthma
   - Eczema
   - Hay fever.

Points to remember
1. What is asthma? Clinically reversible air flow, expiratory obstruction and wheezing.

2. What are the symptoms of asthma? Wheezing; shortness of breath; cough not productive.

Case 4: A patient with respiratory breathlessness
1. Distinguish respiratory from cardiac breathlessness.
2. Functional assessment
   - Distance walked on the flat.
   - How many stairs without stopping?
   - How many pillows at night (PND usually indicates pulmonary oedema but can be respiratory)?
   - Volume of sputum produced may indicate secondary infection.
   - Frequency of acute exacerbations.
   - How many times in hospital, ventilated or home oxygen?
   - Concurrent illness, especially cardiac disease, right heart failure.
   - Drug history: Bronchodilators, steroids, antibiotics, oxygen.
   - Social
     - Heavy smoking
     - Occupational exposure – dust diseases and miners
     - Travel.

Points to remember
1. What is bronchitis? A cough production of sputum for more than 3 months of a year and for more than 2 years in succession.
2. What is emphysema? Permanent enlargement of air spaces and destruction of alveolar walls which is irreversible. Caused by imbalance of proteases and anti-proteases.
3. What is COAD? A clinical diagnosis of bronchospasm supported by a vitalograph leading over time to a physical examination or chest X-ray of emphysema.
4. What is cor pulmonale? A patient with right heart secondary to failure due to respiratory disease.
   - Right heart failure also occurs with heart disease.
   - Left heart failure is always due to heart disease.
5. What is a pink puffer? A patient with type 1 respiratory failure. The patient hyperventilates (low CO_2) to maintain their oxygen tension, hence puffer and pink.
6. What is a blue bloater? Patient with type 2 respiratory failure. The patient allows a degree of hypoxia and the CO_2 to rise, hence blue, cyanosis and CO_2 retention leads to right heart failure and oedema, hence bloater. Absence of clubbing.

Case 5: A patient has thyroid disease is to have a thyroidectomy
There are at least two areas for enquiry:

1. Why is the patient having a thyroid operation?
2. What is the thyroid status? Establish whether the thyroid is hyper-, eu- or hypo-thyroid.

Points to remember
1. Why an operation?
   - Is the swelling causing pressure symptoms on the trachea, larynx or oesophagus? Simple pressure may give difficulty in swallowing or difficulty in breathing. A cancerous change may invade the recurrent laryngeal nerve and cause a reduced or lack of cough.
   - Is there a possibility of cancer? Surgical removal will allow histological examination.
   - Has medical treatment failed to control thyrotoxicosis? Some patients develop an allergic or other adverse reaction to the anti-thyroid drugs.
2. What is the thyroid status? Normal, hypo- or hyper-? Ask about:
   - Weight changes: lost or gain in weight
   - Reaction to the weather tolerant of heat or cold
   - Activity: irritable or sluggish
   - Cardiac symptoms: palpitations may indicate atrial fibrillation, lack of energy and faints may indicate a bradycardia. Heart failure may cause orthopnoea
   - Skin: dry and course with loss of hair or sweating
   - Bowels: diarrhoea or constipation
   - Changes in menstruation
   - Pulse tachycardia and palpitations (tachycardia of anxiety should go during sleep)
3. What drugs may the patient be taking?
   - Carbimazole and propylthiouracil
   - Patients develop rashes and rarely agranulocytosis with carbimazole
   - Before thyroidectomy, iodine is given to reduce the vascularity of the gland.
4. How will you detect and treat a thyrotoxic crisis?
   - A thyroid crisis is equivalent to a hyperadrenergic state.
     - *Increased*: heart rate, BP, temperature, sweating, oxygen consumption may lead to reduced oxygen saturation and increased carbon dioxide production.
     - *Give*: oxygen, IV propranolol 5 mg or other beta blocker to control heart rate, cooling by cold fluids, ice if pyrexial, glucose infusion, IPPV if hypoxia. Hydrocortisone 100 mg 6-hourly. Carbimazole or propylthiouracil or iodine solution may be given by a nasogastric tube.

Case 6: A diabetic patient
1. Duration of disease
2. Current medications
3. Current diet
4. Typical blood sugar levels and how the blood glucose is controlled
5. Pre-existing complications
   - Neuropathy
   - Retinopathy
   - Nephropathy

6. History of: angina, previous MI, claudication, activity limitation, and hypertension
   - Family history
   - Diabetes
   - IHD
   - Hyperlipidaemia
8. Social history
   - Smoking
9. Type of surgery planned
10. Type of anaesthesia.

Case 7: Male patient requiring an inguinal hernia repair

1. What is the first thing you do?
2. What do you want to know about the hernia?
3. What associated questions are relevant?
4. In the general survey the patient says he has a history of snoring at night. What will you do?
5. He also has a runny nose. Will you delay surgery?

Points to remember
1. Introduce yourself, make the patient comfortable.
2. Ask about the presenting problem. Why is he presenting today and not a month ago?
3. Hernia, what are the symptoms ? Is it reducible or obstructed, where is it, how long has it been present? Have there been any operative scars in the area?
4. Inguinal hernias can be associated with the development of an intra-abdominal mass such as carcinoma of the colon. Ask about changes in weight, bowel habit, bleeding PR with symptoms of anaemia, obstruction.
5. Snoring may mean a difficult airway and a difficult intubation. Obstructive sleep apnoea is associated with episodes of nightly hypoxia, which leads, over time, to CVS symptoms such as angina, MI, hypertension and CVA. The longer the night-time hypoxia continues, the more severe the secondary problems. The patient is likely to have postoperative hypoxia warranting HDU care.
6. A coryza is not an indication for delaying surgery. Check that there are no other symptoms or signs of infection. It may be wise to administer an anti-silagogue as such patients often have an irritable airway, produce a lot of secretions and develop laryngospasm.

Case 8: The patient is to have a cataract operation

1. Why are they having the eye surgery? Assess whether the patient can see you or is blind.
2. Which side is the cataract, how long has it been present, how is the other eye?
3. Cataract is associated with problems of old age, diabetes. Is the patient diabetic?

Points to remember

1. How will you start?
2. What do you want to know about the cataract?
3. What other relevance does the cataract have?
4. What systems of the body will you ask about in particular?

   Diabetes is associated with other symptoms of the CVS, renal and neurological systems. Ask about arteriosclerotic symptoms like angina, hypertension, exercise tolerance (may not go far if cannot see), CVA and dizziness. Nocturia. Neuropathy, sympathetic changes like postural hypotension, diarrhoea, changes in the feet of paraesthesia.

   Drugs such as Insulin, GTN, propranolol may affect the diabetes or other hypertensive. The doses of insulin may be controlled by attendance at a general out-patient or special diabetic nurse-run out-patient clinic. Self-testing of own blood or urine. The patient should have a card to show the control.

   Old age is associated with many other diseases, particularly degenerative conditions such as arthritis and previous medical conditions.
5. What drugs might you expect the patient to be taking?

   Multipharmacy: make sure you go into all the drugs the patient is taking and any reactions to drugs.
6. How might the patient be helped in ensuring that their blood glucose control is good?
7. How will you explain about the block?
8. Explain the operative procedure to the patient.
   - The patient will be first on list as a day patient.
   - The patient may be given 300 ml of drink up to 2 hours preoperatively, and may have a diabetic regime of 5–10% glucose infusion 500 ml 6-hourly, with a sliding scale of intramuscular/subcutaneous insulin.
   - The BM stix will be checked every hour while unconscious and 3-hourly when awake.
   - If the operation is performed under local anaesthesia it is possible to rely on an early return to drinking and so possible to miss the morning insulin but give half the morning dose at lunchtime or whole evening dose once drinking again.
   - Explain about cleaning the eye, drops in eye for LA and dilation.
   - Injection while looking straight at ceiling. Feeling of stinging passes off quickly. Eye going numb and not moving with closure of eyelid. Cheek and upper lip numbness. All wear off in a few hours depending on LA used.
   - Risk of haematoma and need for pressure if this happens.

Case 9: You are asked to take a history from a lady for a lower segment caesarian section (LSCS)

A suggested scheme is:

1. Introduce yourself. Then think about:
   - General health

- Nutritional status, build, hydration particularly if nausea and vomiting or urinary frequency
- Increase in weight, a large increase may indicate: polyhydramnios, large baby (diabetes or twins), oedema
- Tiredness, which may indicate anaemia
- LMP and expected date of delivery
- Problems related to this pregnancy, e.g. bleeding, abdominal pain.

2. Past obstetric history
   - Parity
   - Problems of fertility (precious baby)
   - Delivery history.

3. Past medical history
   - Exclude pre-pregnancy problems such as diabetes, heart disease, and respiratory disease
   - Past family history of diabetes, multiple births.

4. Drug history
   - Patient should be taking iron and folic acid supplements
   - Expectation for delivery and any worries
   - Past delivery history
   - Pain relief effective, if not why not, section reason and outcome.

5. Cardiovascular system
   Due to physiological changes in pregnancy ask about:
   - Breathlessness, most women will be breathless from 20 weeks
   - Palpitations, increased heart rate – if excessive think of hyperthyroidism
   - Ankle oedema due to lower limb venous obstruction and lower plasma albumin.

6. Respiration system
   - Observe for dyspnoea, auscultation
   - Airway mouth opening, neck movement, dentition.

7. Nervous system
   - Headache may indicate pre-eclampsia
   - Find out about any nerve defects before the labour, e.g. back pain and sciatica, lateral cutaneous nerve of thigh can get trapped before passing under the inguinal ligament giving a numb thigh.

8. Musculoskeletal system
   - Check the spine for deformity, infection, palpate spaces, if considering an epidural.

9. Renal
   Frequency and nocturia due to:
   - Cystitis infection
   - Low glucose tolerance
   - Proteinuria in pre-eclampsia
   - Pressure of uterus on bladder.

10. GI tract
    - Heartburn: most women have reflux after 30 weeks
    - Nausea and vomiting: morning sickness usually passes off after 18 weeks
    - Constipation and the pregnancy may lead to haemorrhoids.

In taking a history, be alert to medical conditions unrelated to the pregnancy. With a LSCS and pain relief it is relevant to specifically know about conditions like aortic stenosis or cardiomyopathy, bronchospasm, multiple sclerosis and diabetes.

History 1

(Answers on page 25)

You are asked to see a 67 year-old man of for a cystoscopy as a day patient.

Questions

1. Write down what you consider are the important issues in the history that you will ask the patient about – specific to the introduction you have been given.

   Introduce yourself by name, followed by a history of the cystoscopy.

2. What will you ask?

   The patient says he has haematuria.

3. What are the causes of haematuria and what are the follow-up questions that should be asked?

4. How can you differentiate between acute and chronic blood loss?

   Any patient coming for a cystoscopy should have their renal function assessed.

5. What will you ask to assess renal function?

6. What are the relevant points about being a day case?

7. What else should you have asked about?

History 2

(Answers on page 27)

You are asked to see a 79 year-old woman who is on your list for an elective hysterectomy.

Introduce yourself by name.

Questions

1. What issues might be relevant to start with?

   The hysterectomy is for postmenopausal bleeding.

2. What follow up questions does this suggest?

3. How will you assess the amount of blood loss leading to possible anaemia?

   This patient suffers from syncope and has recently been prescribed an ACE inhibitor for hypertension.

4. What do you want to know?

   Does the patient take other drugs?

5. She takes aspirin – why and for what effect?

   The patient now says she is also taking warfarin.

6. Why is she taking warfarin and what difference does this make to your history?

7. Finally, what else will you check for?

History 3
(Answers on page 29)

You are told that at the next station you should take a history from the patient who is to have a thyroidectomy.

Questions

1. How will you start your history taking?

2. What symptoms of thyroid disease will you explore in the history?

   You decide that the symptoms suggest hyperthyroidism.

3. What drug history would you ask about?

4. What associated conditions will you ask about?

   The patient indicates that they had an episode of chest pain and hospital admission 4 weeks ago.

5. What are the possible causes of chest pain and what treatment might follow?

6. What general questions will you ask?

History 4

(Answers on page 30)

You are to take a history from a lady who is to have an arthroscopy.

Questions

1. How will you start?

   The main symptom is a "wheeze or bad chest". The patient might indicate that they have an inhaler.

2. How will you explore this symptom?

   This woman has had a chest problem since childhood.

3. What could be the cause of this scenario? What treatment could have been given that might be related in the history?

   There are many causes of breathlessness.

4. How will you differentiate the types of breathlessness from the history?

5. In what ways may the patient's job have a bearing on the present symptoms?

6. What extra points might be relevant?

History 5 (Answers on page 32)

You are asked to take a relevant history from a patient who has arthritis. She is to have a cholecystectomy.

Start by introducing yourself and asking about her main symptoms.

Questions

1. What are the lines of enquiry you will follow?

2. What types of arthritis may she have and how will you question her to determine which she has?

You decide that this woman has rheumatoid arthritis.

3. What do you need to know about?

4. Which drugs will you enquire about and why?

The operation is to be a cholecystectomy.

5. What symptoms will she have had and what is the differential diagnosis?

The patient indicates that she has diabetes mellitus.

6. What do you need to explore about diabetes?

Answers
History Taking

Answers – History 1

Patient's scenario: Man, with haematuria, has had several cytoscopies for haematuria but recently has had a bigger bleed than usual and comes as a day patient for another cystoscopy.

1. You will want to explore the reasons for the cystoscopy. What symptoms, when did they first occur, how long has he had symptoms for? Also, is he suitable for day care?

2. Check through possible reasons for having a cystoscopy
   a. For poor urine flow – prostatism
   b. Haematuria
   c. Incontinence
   d. Dysuria or pain due to infection
   e. Incontinence – urethral valves.

3. Haematuria
   a. Clotting disorder
      i. Congenital – haemophilia
      ii. Acquired – anticoagulants, bone marrow disorders, and liver disease: does the patient bruise easily or bleed excessively when cut? (Adult causes of a clotting defect? Think of conditions invading the bone marrow. Liver disease linked to a high alcohol intake.)
   b. Infection in bladder or kidney: pain in loin or dysuria
   c. Tumour: bladder, benign papilloma or cancer; renal tract or kidney. Ask about job – dye workers get bladder cancer and pain
   d. Prostate disease: tumour or infection: altered stream, nocturia and frequency, pain dysuria or secondaries give bone pain
   e. Stones: family history, travel to hot climates. Pain in loin, along line of ureter, on passing urine.

   Loss of weight, general ill health or febrile episodes suggest: cancer or infection, may be primary, or secondary to tumour or obstruction to urine flow.

   Check that this is haematuria: from urethra/penis – in the urine? Could it be from the rectum or vagina in a woman?

4. Symptoms of blood loss
   a. How much blood has been lost? Over what period of time? The amount may be reflected in whether the patient felt tiredness or syncope
   b. When did the patient lose blood? Is it a sudden, acute loss or chronic, or acute on chronic?

The effect of acute blood loss depends on the amount of blood loss and the time since the loss. Immediately afterwards there are no changes in the haematocrit but changes in the CVS. A loss of 10% will lead to a tachycardia and vasoconstriction; a loss of 20% blood volume in a fit adult will often not be associated with hypotension. Hypotension becomes apparent with blood loss of 30% of blood volume or more. After a short period of time, haemodilution occurs to recreate the circulating volume. Acute blood loss may be associated with syncope or the sudden onset of angina or breathlessness.

Chronic blood loss will allow time for physiological adjustment, giving a normal circulating volume, normal heart rate and blood pressure but limited exercise tolerance. Chronic blood loss may lead to anaemia and oedema may develop. Consider that you may be asked to explain the different red cell profiles and haematocrits that will occur in acute and chronic blood loss. Acute blood loss will initially show a normal haemoglobin concentration. PCV will depend on the resuscitation fluids. Chronic losses will lead to a low haemoglobin concentration, possible iron deficiency anaemia and a raised reticulocyte count indicating increased turnover of erythrocytes, In contrast, rheumatoid arthritis and chronic renal failure will show a normocytic normochromic anaemia.

5. Concentrating capacity may be reduced. This will present as polyuria and nocturia. Oedema from salt and water retention occurs in chronic renal failure with hypertension. Poor stream and frequency are not necessarily renal symptoms as they may be due to an outflow obstruction.

6. Day care
An assessment of the general state of health ASA 1, 2 or stable 3. Instructions: No food from the night before, drinks up to 2 hours before surgery. Distance from hospital and transport arrangements. Someone to accompany them home and to stay with them for 24 hours. What are the home circumstances, is there a phone at home? Not to drive a car, return to work or do anything that might be affected by the recent drug administration, which could affect their judgement for 24 hours. This could include signing a legal document, operating machinery and cooking. Do they know the arrangements for seeking help, pain relief at home and follow-up?

7. Smoker, alcohol intake, other drugs and allergies, teeth, past history and previous anaesthetics, other symptoms.

Answers – History 2

Patient's scenario: You are an elderly lady with postmenopausal bleeding and atrial fibrillation. You are hypertensive taking an ACE inhibitor, low dose aspirin and warfarin. You are suffering from "fainting attacks", which have become less frequent since starting the warfarin.

This case illustrates the range of problems from which the elderly may suffer. Also the range of drug interactions in the elderly.

1. The reason for the hysterectomy. Problems of the elderly – particularly general health, exercise tolerance and drugs.

2. The causes of bleeding:
   - Carcinoma – weight loss. Clotting disorder
   - Anticoagulant therapy
   - Leukaemia or other marrow dysfunction – bruising.

   How much blood has been lost and when did the symptom start?

   The effect of blood loss: is the patient anaemic with CVS symptoms of breathlessness, angina, oedema and limited exercise tolerance?

3. Ask about the amount of blood loss and for how long – any clots? Ask about general symptoms and, particularly in the elderly, about drug history. Symptoms of weakness, syncope or transient ischaemic episodes, angina, breathlessness and orthopnoea, oedema, exercise limit.

4. It might be logical to link the ACE inhibitor to falls in blood pressure causing syncope if the two started at the same time or if the patient also uses a diuretic. A diuretic such as frusemide causes loss of salt and water. This may lead to thirst, increased water intake, a low serum sodium and aldosterone production. If an ACE inhibitor is added at this stage there is an increased diuresis and a possible fall in blood pressure.

   First think of other casues of syncope, e.g. heart block, anaemia, hypoglycaemia, arteriosclerosis of carotid arteries, other drugs.

   Ask about the possible side-effects of ACE inhibitors: dose, duration of administration. Have there been other treatments for hypertension such as diuretics? ACE inhibitors are used when thiazide diuretics and beta blockers are contraindicated and are particularly indicated in insulin-dependent diabetics. It may be relevant to consider whether the ACE inhibitor was used due to an adverse reaction to another anti-hypertensive drug and what that reaction was. Did the diuretics aggravate the patient's diabetes or gout, or beta blockers aggravate asthma? If a condition like hypertension is mentioned consider the effect it may be having on other organs such as kidneys, eyes and the vessels of heart and brain.

5. Low dose aspirin 75 mg daily is taken as an anti-thrombotic agent to delay arteriosclerosis in angina or to reduce emboli causing TIAs. Larger doses of

600 mg 6-hourly are used for anti-inflammatory pain relief. In this case, check on coagulation status, renal function with ACE inhibitors and aspirin, and possible link to nasal polyps and asthma.

6. Warfarin is probably given for DVT or atrial fibrillation (caused by the hypertension) with evidence of emboli. Has the patient had either diagnosed? It might be aggravating the blood loss.

7. Teeth, allergies, smoker, alcohol.

Answers – History 3

Patient's scenario: You are a patient with a thyroid swelling, clinically thyrotoxic. You are breathless on exertion, atrial fibrillation, on warfarin and aspirin.

1. Start with an introduction and proceed to ask about the present complaint. How long has it been present, when first noticed? Decide if the patient has a mass, which is enlarging; and then symptoms suggesting a thyrotoxic, hypothyroid or euthyroid state.

2. Neck swelling. Are there symptoms of pressure on the airway? This is the upper airway so stridor implies tracheal narrowing. Infiltration into the surrounding tissue may occur with cancer, not a goitre. Hoarseness by pressure on the recurrent laryngeal nerve implies carcinoma of the thyroid.

   Hyperthyroid symptoms: hyperactivity, sweating, palpitations particularly in the elderly, loss of weight with increased appetite, diarrhoea and heat intolerance. Signs of tremor, warm peripheries, pretibial oedema and exophthalmos. Alterations in menstruation.

   Hypothyroid symptoms: weight gain, dry thin hair and hair loss, gruff or deep-toned voice, constipation, cold intolerance and a slowing of mental activity. Bradycardia and pericardial effusions may give rise to breathlessness.

3. The patient may be taking carbimazole. Carbimazole is commonly used to inhibit the formation of thyroid hormones. Be sure there are no side-effects: nausea, rashes, pruritus, jaundice and, rarely, life-threatening blood dyscrasia presenting as a sore throat. Propylthiouracil is used when there are side-effects to carbimazole. Propranolol may be used for supraventricular tachycardias associated with hyperthroid states.

   About 5 days before surgery, iodine is given to reduce the vascularity of the gland.

4. There is a link between hyperthyroidism and other autoimmune conditions such as pernicious anaemia and myasthenia gravis. Symptoms of muscle weakness and lid lag. Anaemia might give CVS symptoms and fatigue. Where does the patient come from? Goitres are more common in mountainous areas where iodine is deficient in the water.

5. There might be: palpitations from atrial fibrillation, a thyrotoxic crisis, a myocardial infarction or conditions unrelated to the thyrotoxicosis, such as a chest infection, pulmonary embolism, oesophagitis, or herpes zoster. Check that this was chest pain and not an abdominal pain.

   It is important to ask about possible complications of a myocardial infarction such as: angina, palpitations, breathlessness and oedema.

   Drugs: aspirin 75 mg or more daily, beta blocker, GTN, anticoagulants, calcium channel blocker.

6. Previous anaesthetics, smoking, alcohol, other drugs and allergies, teeth, veins and family history.

Answers – History 4

Patient's scenario: You are a patient with bronchiectasis (but would not tell the examining doctor this diagnosis unless specifically asked: "do you have bronchiectasis?"). You are working and reasonably active. For arthroscopy as a day patient. Wheeze, sputum, bronchodilators. Measles as a child and several periods in hospital in teens with postural drainage. You had a lobectomy 10 years ago.

1. Two issues to start with:
   a. Why the arthroscopy? What is the problem, e.g. pain? How long has it been a problem, what caused it?
   b. General health – what are the main symptoms; drugs, past history and operations, social history?
   Five minutes goes very quickly so do not get fixed or dwell on just one problem. At this stage you know the reason for the operation and at least one symptom.

2. Ask about the chest symptoms in a systematic way, otherwise you may jump to the wrong diagnosis.
   a. Cough, is it productive?
   b. Sputum colour and how much? Chronic bronchitis is a cough productive of sputum for more than 3 months of the year and for more than 2 years in succession.
   c. Haemoptysis – could be chronic bronchitis, carcinoma, or tuberculosis.
   d. Wheeze. When is it worse – morning or evening; what aggravates it – allergies; any hospital admissions?
   e. Shortness of breath at rest or on exercise. How much is the exercise tolerance? Wheeze and breathlessness are symptoms of respiratory and cardiovascular diseases.
   f. Pain. How long have the symptoms been a problem. Does the patient have an acute or chronic problem?
   Differential diagnosis:

   - Acute: pneumonia, pneumothorax (unlikely in an examination).
   - Chronic: bronchitis, bronchiectasis, asthma, restrictive disease following injury, gassing or fractures, occupational disease following mining, carcinoma. Sarcoidosis affects women with fatigue and weight loss; tuberculosis may induce night sweats, haemoptysis and weight loss.
   - Haemoptysis: think carcinoma, bronchitis, TB, bronchiectasis, coagulation disorder, left ventricular failure if frothy.
   - The inhalers may be salbutamol or a steroid. Is the patient (or have they been) taking systemic steroids?

3. Childhood symptoms suggest a congenital problem or childhood illness, trauma.

   Cystic fibrosis. Bronchiectasis following a childhood pneumonia may follow illness such as measles or whooping cough, or an inhaled foreign body (peanuts), childhood asthma.

Ask about: Treatment with antibiotics, steroids and bronchodilators. Bronchodilators are used for conditions other than asthma. Postural drainage. Operations to remove part of the lung which is diseased. Treatment for tuberculosis or sarcoidosis.

4. Breathlessness can be respiratory or cardiovascular in origin. Breathless upright or with exercise implies limited gaseous exchange either due to reduced cardiac or respiratory function.

   Respiratory breathlessness – ask about "wheeze" rather than asthma which is one specific type of wheeze. Alveolar and small airway obstruction will first cause an expiratory wheeze. Upper airway obstruction first gives an inspiratory wheeze. Asthma is associated with reversible airway obstruction, which varies in severity during the day, usually worse in the morning. Chronic obstructive airways disease gives rise to a non-reversible wheeze.

   Cardiovascular breathlessness due to congestion in the lung with oedema will get worse with lying down, suggesting: orthopnoea, or paroxysmal nocturnal dyspnoea (PNI). PND suggest pulmonary oedema but can be asthma. The wheeze of pulmonary oedema is more permanent than a respiratory wheeze, may be relieved by diuretics and failure will give frothy sputum.

   While talking you may notice signs of breathlessness, cyanosis, hand tremor and clubbing, but it is not part of your task to examine the patient in the history taking station.

5. Miners, or workers with asbestos or in a dusty atmosphere can develop restrictive lung diseases, including asbestosis. Farmers working in damp barns get farmer's lung.

   Hobbies: keeping pigeons can cause an allergic alveolitis.

   Smoker and lung cancer.

6. In a person with a chest complaint consider: smoking, do they take regular antibiotics, do they get influenza immunisation in the winter? You would not want to operate in the winter. Have they required hospital admission and ventilator support?

   General health, teeth, alcohol intake.

Answers – History 5

Patient's scenario: Arthritis – lead to diagnosis of rheumatoid rather than osteoarthritis. Operation – cholecystectomy for abdominal pain, might not be gall stones. Diabetic on oral hypoglycaemic and diet.

1. Take your lead from the introductory statement. The type of arthritis and the symptoms leading to the cholecystectomy. How long has the patient had symptoms, when did they start?

2. Osteoarthritis, rheumatoid arthritis (RA), ankylosing spondylitis or linked to psoriasis, polymyalgia rheumatica, gout, or a connective tissue disorder?

   Ask about duration of illness and possible injury. Types of joints affected. Pain, type, when worse and what makes it easier.

   Osteoarthritis pain is in the knees, hips, hands, aggravated by movement, eased by rest, morning stiffness, large joint deformity. Osteoarthritis often affects a single joint and may follow a traumatic insult.

   Rheumatoid arthritis causes pain in the small joints of hands and feet, with morning stiffness but improving with activity. About 25% of patients have only one joint affected, general fatigue and malaise common, other organs affected. Non-weight-bearing joints are more involved with RA, which is usually a polyarthropathy affecting joints in a symmetrical pattern.

   Osteo- and rheumatoid arthritis are both familial. Single joint involvement in gout.

3. Neck movement. Atlanto-axial subluxation can give rise to serious neurological signs. Mouth opening may be limited by temperomandibular joint limitation of movement. Renal function anaemia, lung function.

   Anaemia is common. Thrombocytosis is linked to the activity of the disease.

   Lungs: pleural effusions, and small airway disease. The skin can be affected by a vasculitis which leads to ischaemia and gangrene of fingers and toes.

   Possible arteritis with rheumatoid and autoimmune diseases may involve: kidneys, respiratory or cardiovascular systems giving breathlessness. Sight is affected in Sjögren's syndrome – dry eyes or scleritis in RA and auto-immune disease, steroid effect of psoriasis.

4. Analgesics, RA specific agents and steroids and for how long? Steroids may need supplementation around the time of operation. Steroid effects: on skin and subcutaneous tissue, hypertension, diabetic state, osteoporotic fractures, mental effect paranoia or depression, proximal muscle wasting, peptic ulceration exacerbation. NSAIDs. Agents to suppress the disease process such as Gold, Penicillamine, Azothioprine.

5. Differentiate pain above the diaphragm: myocardial infarction, pneumonia, hiatus hernia; below the diaphragm: cholecystitis, peptic ulcer, diabetes porphyria, bowel disorders such as irritable bowel syndrome, inflammatory bowel disease. Has the patient been jaundiced?

6. Diabetes. Diet and drugs – which ones and for how long? How well controlled is the diabetes? Urine or blood sampling; at home or special clinic, role of diabetic specialist nurse. Diabetes affects many organs. Ask about: features of arteriosclerosis, angina, transient ischaemic episodes, angina, claudication. Renal function – kidney infection and glomerular impairment and vascular changes similar to hypertensive changes.

Neurological changes will affect 80% of diabetics. The legs may be affected by a sensory or autonomic neuropathy leading to postural hypotension causing syncope on standing. Autonomic neuropathy is common affecting the bladder function and incontinence. Ask about paraesthesia, numbness or burning sensations, diarrhoea.

Eye sight is affected by cataracts and new vessels growing on to the iris and retina, and a sixth nerve palsy.

Weight loss.

The foot is at risk from ischaemia, ulcers and infection. Leg pain and ischaemia may limit exercise making it difficult to assess the severity of cardiovascular or respiratory disease.

Arterial occlusion symptoms may also present as angina, claudication or stroke.

PHYSICAL EXAMINATION

2

Time is limited to 5 minutes and therefore you must have a method and practise it with someone looking on to check that it is correct. In reality, time is limited for preoperative assessment so it is not unrealistic to expect a candidate to examine a system in 5 minutes.

There are three aspects to practice for an examination.

1. Perform a logical examination.
2. Make deductions as you proceed.
3. Tell the examiner what you are doing, what you are looking for and what you have found as you proceed.

Specific examinations to practise.

1. Airway assessment
2. Respiratory system
3. Arterial pulse
4. Central venous pressure.
5. Blood pressure measurement.
6. Praecordium
7. Cranial nerves
8. CNS apart from the cranial nerves
9. Trauma patient/Glasgow Coma Scale
10. An obstetric patient.

Physical Examination stations can involve:

Part of a patient
- Antecubital fossa
- The wrist
- Airway

System or part of a system
- Pulse
- Precordium
- Blood pressure.

Remember

You must have a method; practise performing a routine examination of each system and part of the body and do it in a finite time.

You should read the briefing note about the station in the examination hall, which you will find on display before meeting the patient. Mentally prepare what you will do.

There will be an examiner who will introduce you to the patient and will then observe your performance and allocate marks according to standard guidelines.

The examiner may talk to you but you should not wait for them to do so before beginning the task that has been indicated. You may find it helpful to explain what you are doing as you proceed. Rather than standing and inspecting say what you are looking at and what you have found.

Prepare yourself with at least a stethoscope.

When you examine the respiratory or cardiovascular systems use the same routine.

1. Inspection
2. Palpitation
3. Percussion
4. Auscultation.

Always start by introducing yourself to the patient and briefly explain what you want the patient to do.

Physical examination 1   (Answers on page 57)

AIRWAY assessment
You are asked to examine the airway and explain each procedure.

Questions
1. What will you look for on general inspection?

2. How can you test the nose?

3. What will you look for in and around the mouth?

4. How will you assess neck movement?

5. Describe the Mallampati airway classification.

6. Describe the Wilson risk score.

7. What is the prayer sign?

8. What tests may be used when the airway is difficult?

Physical examination 2 *(Answers on page 60)*

Respiratory system

You are asked to demonstrate how to examine the respiratory system.

Questions

1. General inspection. What should this include?

2. How should the chest be examined?

3. What are the common breath sounds?

4. What tests can be performed at the bedside?

5. Describe the findings that might be present in
   a. emphysema
   b. right apical fibrosis.

Self-test: Respiratory system *(Answers on page 64)*

This is another test of your technique for examining the respiratory system.

Questions

1. What position should the patient be in?

2. Start by inspection. What are you looking for?

3. Palpate the trachea position and the apex position. Palpate the chest wall and movement with respiration. What are you feeling for and what may it mean?

4. Percussion. Think how you will do this with the least fuss. Slow practitioners are those who repeat everything. So get into the habit of placing the hand on to the chest wall and tapping once only in each position. Three taps takes three times as long and if you train your ear three taps will give you no more information than one tap – percuss at the apex and bases right and left. What changes may be detected?

5. Tactile fremitus or vibration. Place the ulnar side of the hand against the chest wall and ask the patient to say "99". What does an increase mean?

6. Auscultation. What will this detect?

7. What simple bedside tests can be performed of lung function?

Physical examination 3 *(Answers on page 66)*

Arterial pulse

You are asked to examine the arterial pulse.

Start by examining the radial, brachial or carotid, whichever you are familiar with unless asked specifically to examine a particular pulse. Do not forget to check the other side and offer to examine the femoral pulses.

Questions

1. Which characteristics of the normal pulse can you describe?

2. What is sinus arrhythmia and what causes it?

3. What is the character of the pulse in aortic stenosis, thyrotoxicosis and asthma?

4. What is the pulse pressure? What causes an increase in pulse pressure?

(Answers on page 69)

Self-test: Taking the pulse

Questions

1. What can you tell by examining the radial pulse?

2. Demonstrate the features of a collapsing pulse.

3. Name at least three conditions in which the pulse is collapsing.

4. Demonstrate a modified Allen's test.

5. What would a positive modified Allen's test be?

6. What did Allen originally describe the test for?

7. What is pulsus alternans?

8. What is pulsus paradoxus?

9. Name three complications of radial arterial catheterisation.

Physical examination 4 *(Answers on page 70)*

Central venous pressure measurement

- Introduce yourself and explain what you want to do.
- Expose the neck properly.
- Position the patient 45° to the horizontal and head turned to one side.

Questions

1. Outline an order for the examination.

2. How does the waveform change in disease?

3. How would you differentiate between venous and arterial pulsations in the neck?

4. How do vascular disorders affect the venous pressure?

Physical examination 5 *(Answers on page 71)*

Blood pressure measurement
You are asked to measure the blood pressure and explain the technique.

Questions
1. Blood pressure reading. How will you measure the blood pressure?

2. Which arm will you measure it in and why?

3. What is the name of the sounds?

4. When is systolic pressure taken?

5. When is diastolic pressure taken?

6. What are the landmarks of the brachial artery as it enters the antecubital fossa, where the blood pressure is usually taken?

7. What size of cuff bladder should be used?

8. What is the effect of using a narrow cuff on an obese patient?

9. What is the effect of reading the blood pressure in the foot when the patient is supine?

Self-test: Blood pressure measurement

(Answers on page 73)

Questions

1. What happens to the BP when standing?

2. What is orthostatic hypotension?

3. What is a DINAMP?

4. What is the MOA of a DINAMP?

5. When is systolic and diastolic pressure taken using a DINAMP?

Calibration

6. Give examples of devices, which gives absolute values and others that, need calibrating.

7. How is each calibrated?

8. What is drift and gain?

Physical examination 6 *(Answers on page 74)*

Praecordium
You are asked to examine the praecordium.

Questions
1. What is the praecordium?

2. What is the first thing you do?

3. What routine should be followed?

Self-test: Cardiovascular system

(Answers on page 77)

You are asked to examine the cardiovascular system.

Start by making sure that the patient is comfortable, undressed to the waist, and lying at about an angle of 45° to the horizontal.

Start with inspection of:

- Hands
- Pulses
- Blood pressure
- Lips or conjunctiva
- Face
- Neck
- Sacrum and ankles
- Thorax.

Questions

1. What can be learnt from examining the hands?

2. What can be learnt from the pulse?

3. Blood pressure. If the blood pressure is high what will you examine?

4. What does cyanosis mean?

5. What may the face show relevant to the CVS?

6. Look at the neck and the jugular pulse.
   a. How do you differentiate the venous from the carotid pulse?
   b. What are the surface markings of the internal jugular vein?
   c. Describe the normal venous pulse in the neck?
   d. Under what circumstances do you get prominent v wave?
   e. How would you fill the neck veins to demonstrate their presence?

7. The sacrum and ankles. How does oedema form?

8. Thorax. Inspect for shape and pulsations. Palpate the precordium.
   What is the normal position of the apex beat?
   What would suggest left or right ventricular enlargement? Some murmurs are palpable as thrills.

9. Auscultation for heart sounds and murmurs. Try to make a diagnosis before placing the stethoscope on the chest from the inspection and signs already found. What will be the cause of a systolic or a diastolic murmur?

Physical examination 7

Cranial nerves

Nervous system can be divided into cranial nerves, intellectual functions and the peripheral nervous system.

Concentrate on the tests in bold type.

1. **Olfactory**
   - Assess patency of airway, identify standard odours. This cranial nerve has little importance.
2. **Optic nerve**
   - The only nerve that can be seen – **look at the retina** – haemorrhages and exudates occur in hypertension and diabetes mellitus.
   - Assess visual acuity. With spectacles near and far vision in each eye.
   - **Visual fields.** Sit opposite the patient and ask them to look straight ahead at your nose while you look at their nose. Hold your hands at the level of your eyes, such that you can just see a finger to the left and right. Move the fingers inwards until the patient can see the movement. When the patient can see both fingers, move the fingers together to test for visual inattention. A pituitary lesion will produce a bitemporal hemianopia. Draw the optic nerves, chiasma and tracts and explain how this happens.
   - Colour vision test with colour plates.
   - **Pupils** reaction to light (from a light brought in from the side) and accommodation – constriction as the eye focuses on a near object (a light shone near to the eye).
   - The pupils in both eyes will normally constrict when one eye is tested = a consensual light reflex.

3. **Third cranial nerve**
   - All the extra-ocular muscles except lateral rectus and superior oblique. A third nerve palsy leads to the eye being DOWN and OUT, ptosis, mydriasis, loss of light and accommodation reflexes.
   - The commoner causes of this problem are idiopathic, intracranial aneurysms, head injury, multiple sclerosis, hypertension and diabetes.

4. **Trochlear nerve**
   - Supplies superior oblique (SO_4).

5. **Trigeminal nerve**
   - **Sensory** from face up to the crown, taste to anterior two-thirds of tongue, and mouth mucosa. Corneal reflex.
   - Motor to masseter muscles, temporalis.

Test: **Jaw reflex** by tapping mandible with mouth open.

Touch face with cotton wool and pinprick or cold. **Corneal reflex** with cotton wool.

Shut mouth, clench teeth – masseter muscle; try to close mouth against resistance – pterygoids.

6. Abducens nerve
- Supplies lateral rectus (LR_6).

7. Facial nerve
- Motor to muscles of facial expression.
- Sensory from anterior two-thirds of tongue.
- Forehead muscle innervated for both sides of cortex so spared in upper motor neurone lesion CVA. A lower motor neurone lesion (Bell's palsy) paralyses the whole of one side of the face.

Test: **Screw eyes up, show teeth, smile.**

8a. Vestibular nerve
- Concerned with balance.

Test: **nystagmus** when sudden movements are made like rolling from one side to the other or from lying to sitting.

8b. Cochlear nerve
- Hearing.

Rinne's test: **Place tuning fork on mastoid until the sound fades then place over external meatus and the noise should still be heard. Shows air conduction better than bone conduction.**

Weber test: **Place tuning fork on the centre of the forehead. The sound is heard best on the side of the diseased ear. Or the normal ear with nerve deafness.**

9. Glossopharyngeal nerve
- Sensory to posterior third of tongue.
- Motor muscles of swallowing.

Test: Ask the patient to exhibit **swallow and gag reflex** by touching a spatula against the back of the mouth.

10. Vagus
Test: Ask patient to exhibit **cough, vocalise, gag and palate reflexes.**

11. Accessory nerve
- Motor to trapezius and sternomastoid.

Test: **Shrug the shoulders, turn head against resistance.**

12. Hypoglossal nerve
- Motor to tongue.

Test: **Put tongue straight out.**

Self-test 1: Cranial nerves   *(Answers on page 79)*

You are asked to examine the cranial nerves.

At each stage note how you will make the examination, or do it with a patient or colleague and then check against the relevant answer paragraph.

Examine the cranial nerves.

Questions
How will you test the function of the:

1. First nerve: **Olfactory nerve.**

2. Second nerve: **Optic nerve.**

3. Third, fourth and sixth nerves: **Oculomotor, Trochlear and Abducent.**

4. Fifth cranial nerve: **Trigeminal nerve.**

5. Seventh nerve: **Facial nerve.**

6. Eighth nerve: **Auditory and Vestibular nerves.**

7. Ninth nerve: **Glossopharyngeal nerve.**

8. Tenth nerve: **Vagus nerve.**

9. Eleventh nerve: **Accessory nerve.**

10. Twelfth nerve: **Hypoglossal nerve.**

Self-test 2: Cranial nerves   *(Answers on page 82)*

Questions

1. What changes might the eye show in diabetes?

2. If there is bi-temporal field loss where is the lesion?

3. What are the features of Horner's syndrome and which nerve(s) is(are) involved?

4. What does a unilateral ptosis indicate?

5. An inability to bite properly may be a lesion of which nerve? Which muscle is involved?

6. Loss of taste to the anterior two-thirds of the tongue involves which nerves?

7. If the conduction is heard best in the right ear when the tuning fork is placed on the forehead but the patient complains of deafness in the right ear what is the problem?

8. How would you test the functioning of the 9th cranial nerve?

9. What symptom may indicate a 10th nerve palsy?

10. Which muscle movements are tested for 11th nerve function?

Physical examination 8

Central nervous system (not cranial nerves)

High functions
- Level of consciousness, orientation **self-knowledge, time, place**
- Memory recent and long-term.
- General intelligence.
- Speech and language.
- Gait and walking co-ordination, weaknesses.
- Establish which is the **dominant hand** as the muscles may be better developed on that side.

Sensory function
- Test skin in distribution of **dermatomes and peripheral nerves.**
- **Pain** with cold or pinprick.
- Temperature with cold metal.
- Light touch with cotton wool or finer touch.
- Joint, **position and vibration sense.** Close eyes and move a joint. Place tuning fork on bone should sense a tingling sensation.

Motor function
- **Look at muscles for wasting,** fasciculation, involuntary movements.
- **Tone.** Reduced – flaccid in a lower motor nerve lesion. Increased – spasticity with an upper motor nerve lesion. Pyramidal – clasp knife (stiff at the start of extension like a penknife opening) with brisk reflexes. Extra-pyramidal – lead pipe (stiff throughout the range of movement), combined with a tremor becomes cogwheel. Take the flexed arm and feel how it extends.
- **Power.** Compare sides.
- Fine movements and co-ordination.
- **Reflexes of tendons**
  - Arm supinator C5/6, biceps C5/6, triceps C6/7.
  - Leg knee – patella L4, ankle - Achilles S1 (dorsiflexion of hallux L5).
  - Plantar reflex. Stimulation of side of foot produces plantar flexion.
    - An extensor response (Babinski sign) due to upper motor neurone lesion.
- **Rapid movement.** Tap table rapidly, finger nose test, run heel up shin.

Gait
Romberg's test: Stand erect, heels together, eyes closed. Does the patient lean to one side? Repeat standing on one foot.

Ask patient to walk away and then back.

Self-test 1: CNS

(Answers on page 83)

You are asked to examine the nervous system, apart from the cranial nerves.

Questions

1. What tests will you perform of brain stem and cerebellar function?

The peripheral nervous system is divided into:
- Efferent – motor function
- Afferent – sensory input
- Autonomic nervous system both efferent and afferent.

2. How will you test motor function?

3. How will you test sensory funtion?

4. How do you perform straight leg raising, sciatic and femoral stretch tests? What does pain during these tests mean?

(Answers on page 85)

Self-test 2: CNS

Questions

1. What position does the arm take up following an upper brachial plexus palsy such as might occur from traction while lying on the operating table?

2. Which nerve roots are affected if the triceps reflexes are reduced?

3. What position does the arm assume in a palsy of the radial, median, and ulnar nerves? What is the distribution of the loss of sensation in each case?

4. If there is a sensory level below the clavicles and normal arm function, at what level is the lesion likely to be?

5. A sensory level at the umbilicus suggests a lesion at which spinal root?

6. If the patient is unable to dorsiflex the hallux, which nerve root may be affected?

7. Numbness on the medial calf can be due to which nerve defect, and which dermatome?

8. Name three causes of Parkinsonism.

9. The treatment for idiopathic Parkinsonism involves which drugs?

10. Name three conditions leading to a loss of a knee jerk.

Physical examination 9 *(Answers on page 86)*

Trauma patient/Glasgow Coma Scale

Questions

1. How would you assess a road traffic accident victim? What is the first stage of the examination?

2. How would you assess the CNS?

An obstetric patient

You are asked to examine a lady for LSCS

Questions

1. How will you start?

2. What general examination will you make?

3. What changes can you demonstrate when you examine the following systems?

a. CVS

b. RS

c. Abdomen

d. CNS

e. Musculoskeletal

f. Renal

Answers
Physical Examination

Answers – Physical examination 1

General inspection

1. You should look for specific findings that may indicate a difficult airway

- Short, muscular neck
- Morbid obesity
- Prominent incisors
- Receding chin
- Inability to open mouth
- Injuries to face, neck, or chest must be evaluated to assess their contribution to airway compromise
- Neck masses
- Large breasts.

Head and neck examination

2. Nose:

- The patency of the nares or presence of a deviated septum should be determined by occluding one and then the other nostril and asking the patient which side permits easier breathing.

3. Mouth:

- Mouth opening
  - Patient should be able to open the mouth at least three finger breadths
- Teeth
  - Poor dentition
  - Loose teeth
- Tongue
  - Marcroglossia is seen in a variety of congenital syndromes.
  - Movement at the tempero-mandibular joint.

4. Neck:

- Cervical spine mobility
  - Patients should be able to touch their chin to their chest and extend their neck as far posteriorly as possible. Patient is sitting. One finger on the occiput and another on the chin. The chin finger should rise higher than the occiput finger.
- Thyro-mental distance
  - The distance from the lower border of the mandible to the thyroid

notch with the neck fully extended and the patient in the supine position
- Distance less than 6.0 cm may predict difficult intubation.

Airway classification

5. The Mallampati classification.
Assessment is made with

- The patient *sitting* upright
- Head in *neutral* position
- The *mouth open* as wide as possible
- The tongue protruded maximally.

The following structures are visible

Class I – Hard palate, soft palate, uvula and tonsillar pillars
Class II – Hard palate, soft palate, uvula
Class III – Hard palate, soft palate
Class IV – Hard palate.

6. Wilson risk score (Br J Anaesthesia 1988;61:211–216)
Five useful risk factors, max 10 points. A score of 4 or more predicts 75% of difficult intubations.

- Weight: 0 = < 90 kg, 1 = 90–110 kg, 2 = > 110 kg.
- Head and neck movement: 0 = above 90°, 1 = about 90°, 2 = below 90°
- Jaw movement, measured by inter-incisor gap (IG) and subluxation (SL): 0 = IG equal or over 5 cm or SL 0, 1 = IG under 5 and SL 0, 2 = IG < 5 cm and SL < 0
- Receding mandible: 0 = normal, 1 = moderate, 2 = severe
- Buck teeth: 0 = normal, 1 = moderate, 2 = severe

7. Prayer sign

- Asking the patient to place both palms flat together. Failure of the palms to be flat together suggests arthritic changes in the hands and neck.

8. Test when a difficult airway is suspected.

- Cervical spine films. Look for a wide anterior space > 5 mm between the axis and the odontoid peg. Flexion and extension films may show little neck movement or subluxation and the degree of disease state, e.g. rheumatoid arthritis
- Chest X-ray. Look for the position and width of the trachea and superior mediastinal tumours
- CT scan of the neck
- Arterial blood gases. Gives a base line. Indicates extreme respiratory failure
- Pulmonary function tests

- Laryngoscopy
  - Direct
  - Indirect
  - Fibreoptic.

Answers – Physical examination 2

1. General examination of hands, face, neck.
Examine the patient by looking at the:
a. Hands
- *Nicotine* on fingers.
- *Clubbing.* The commoner causes are: congenital; respiratory – sign of bronchial cancer, chronic lung sepsis such as occurs in bronchiectasis and lung abscess, fibrosing alveolitis, asbestosis, cardiac – cyanotic congenital heart disease (Fallot's tetralogy), infective endocarditis; gut – ulcerative colitis, Crohn's disease, liver cirrhosis.
- *Cyanosis.* Peripheral cyanosis is a localized circulation problem of the fingers or toes. Central cyanosis of the mucosa of the conjunctiva, inside the mouth and tongue implies respiratory of cardiac disease with a large right to left shunt. More than 5 g of deoxygenated haemoglobin is entering the systemic circulation.
- *Signs of hypercarbia*
  - Warm hands
  - Dilated veins
  - Coarse tremor/flap
  - Sweating hands
  (also tachycardia, reduced consciousness)
- Pallor
- Pulse (bounding pulse)
b. Face
- Eye – papilloedema
- Tongue – central cyanosis
c. Neck
- Lymphadenopathy
- Trachea: it is midline or deviated to one side?
- Distended neck veins
d. Sputum – amount and colour.

2. Chest
Rest the patient comfortably in the bed at 45°. It is often best to examine the front of the chest and then ask the patient to sit forward to examine the back rather than see-saw backwards and forwards. If you use this approach do not forget to allow time for examining the back.

Count the respiratory rate.

Inspection
Chest wall – look for

- Deformities of the chest wall
- Operation scars
- Asymmetry

Breathing patterns – note

- Rate
- Depth
- Regularity.

Palpation

- Start palpation by feeling for the position of the *trachea*. Should be central above the sternal notch.
- The position of the *apex beat*. 1 cm medial to the mid-clavicular line, 5th intercostal space.
- Palpate the chest for local *tenderness*.
- *Chest expansion*: to determine if both sides of the chest move equally. Put the fingers of both your hands as far round the chest as possible and then bring the thumbs together in the midline but keep the thumbs off the chest wall.

  The patient is asked to take a deep breath in. The chest wall, by moving outwards, moves the fingers outwards and the thumbs are in turn distracted away from the midline.
- *Vocal fremitus*: this is performed by placing the flat of your hand on the chest and asking the patient to count one, two, three.

Vibrations are felt by hand.

Percussion

Aim is to detect the resonance or hollowness of the chest.

- Percuss with the middle finger of one hand against the middle phalanx of the middle finger of the other laid flat on the chest. The finger should strike at right angles. Practise making one tap in each position and listening to the note produced. Repeated tapping wastes time and does not give more information.
- Percuss both sides of the chest at top, middle, lower segments. Compare sides and the front with the back.
- Percuss the level of the diaphragm from above downwards.
- Dull in collapse, consolidation, fibrosis. Very dull over fluid. Dullness will usually be associated with a shift in the trachea.
- Hyper-resonance in emphysema, pneumothorax.

By this stage you should have formulated a differential diagnosis.

Auscultation

- Before listening, ask patient to cough up any sputum. A bronchitis patient will have added crackle sounds which clear after a cough.
- Use the bell of the stethoscope.
- Listen at the top, middle, bottom of both sides of the chest and then in the axilla and do not forget front and the back of the chest.
- Ask the patient to take large breaths through their open mouth. Normal breathing is silent.

Listen for:

* Breath sounds:
Normal or vesicular breath sounds due to turbulent air flowing in the larger airways. The noise is transmitted to the surface through normal lung tissue. The sound is louder in inspiration and fades quickly in expiration. These sounds are reduced bilaterally (if obesity) or unilaterally (if fluid or air in a pneumothorax) prevents the transmission. There is less sound from a collapsed lung or in hypoventilation.

  Bronchial sounds occur over the trachea and, when solid, lung tissue transmits noises better. Higher frequencies and loudness are not lost so the sounds are harsher and inspiration sounds as loud and as long as expiration. There is a pause between inspiration and expiration. This occurs over consolidation, fibrosis and collapse.

* Added sounds.

3. There are three common types of added sounds – crackles, wheezes and rubs.

   * Crackles (crepitations) due to turbulent flow as air passes through airways that suddenly open or as air passes intermittently through secretions.
   * Wheezing (rhonchi) indicates constricted air passages where turbulence is increased. Maximum on expiration. Occur on inspiration in the larynx and trachea and when narrowing is severe. No sound indicates very severe spasm.
   * Pleural rub.
   A coarse crackle due to the inflamed visceral and parietal pleura rubbing against each other. Occurs with infection, trauma and infarction.

   Vocal resonance.

   Normally no high pitched voice sounds are transmitted to the surface. When the conditions for bronchial breathing exist, then whispered voice will be transmitted to the surface. This can be felt as tactile vocal fremitus or heard as whispering petriloquy.

   Ask the patient to repeat "99" whilst listening to chest in the same areas as auscultation.

4. At the bed side

   * Blow out a flame at 15 cm with the mouth open.
   * Hold the breath for 30 seconds.
   * Expiration should be completed in less than 6 seconds (normally under 2 seconds).
   * Vitalograph. Ask the patient to take a maximum breath in and then breathe forcefully out.
   * Peak flow. A normal value should be between 400 and 500 l/min for a young adult.

5. Check
   a. Emphysema
      Barrel shaped chest, ribs horizontal, signs of expiratory pursing of lips
      to increase PEEP. Hyper-resonant chest wall bilaterally, reduced air
      entry, crackles thoughout the lung with possible wheeze.
   b. Apical fibrosis
      Flattening of chest wall at apex, trachea pulled over to affected side,
      dull to percussion, reduced air entry over the apex. Bronchial breathing
      at apex.

Answers – Self-test: Respiratory system

1. Sitting comfortably at a 45° incline.

2. Central cyanosis of the mucosa inside the lips and peripheral cyanosis in the fingers. Central cyanosis suggests respiratory failure or a cardiac lesion with a right to left shunt, whereas peripheral cyanosis may be a local disorder of the hand.

   Count the respiratory rate.

   Hands for clubbing. A sign of bronchial cancer, chronic sepsis of the lung such as bronchiectasis. The nicotine staining of the smoker.

   Look for abnormalities of the chest wall. Flattening of part of the chest wall may indicate underlying collapse, fibrosis or past surgery.

   The hyper-expansion of emphysema. Sputum: amount and colour.

3. A shift in the trachea away from the mid line indicates underlying disease. Is it being pushed by tumour or pulled by fibrosis? A shift in the apex beat may mean a shift in the mediastinum.

   Hold your hands against the chest wall with the thumb tips touching over the sternum and watch the movement of breathing. Does one side move more than the other? Repeat at the back of the chest or wait until the patient is sat forward to examine all of the chest from the back, having completed the examination from the front.

4. Percussion leading to resonance suggests hyper-inflation as in emphysema, a pneumothorax – unlikely in the examination. Dullness suggests collapse, consolidation or fibrosis. Very dull suggests fluid in an effusion. Dullness will usually be associated with a shift in the trachea to that side.

5. Tactile fremitus increases in conditions in which the sound is transmitted easily to the periphery of the lung, e.g. consolidation.

6. By now you should be expecting to hear something different if it exists. Your examination up to this point should give you a good idea of where the problem is and what you might hear.

   Ask the patient to breathe through the open mouth, otherwise under normal circumstances little will be heard. Normal breathing is silent. You are listening for increased or reduced sounds, and then extra sounds of wheeze or pulmonary secretions, oedema etc. Air sounds will be reduced if the lung is poorly ventilated as in collapse, lung fibrosis, effusion or pneumothorax.

   Bronchial breathing occurs due to the transmission of bronchial or tracheal sounds that is an equal inspiratory and expiratory sound directly to the periphery through consolidated, collapsed or fibrosed lung. Bronchial breathing is an equal quality of sound during inspiration and expiration.

   Added sounds are unlikely in the examination hall as pulmonary oedema and pneumonia patients will not be fit enough to come. So the bronchitic with his cough may have added sounds but check whether they stay after a cough.

7. The healthy patient can blow a flame out at 15 cm with an open mouth and hold their breath for 30 seconds.

Do you know how to use a simple vitalograph or peak flow meter? Simple peak flow meters are made available to patients with asthma to test their own function.

Ask the patient to take a maximum breath in and blow out into the device as quickly as possible.

A normal value should be a PEFR between 400 and 500 l/min for a young adult.

Answers – Physical examination 3

1. Pulse characteristics

Rate
a. The radial pulse at the wrist is generally used.
b. The rate of the pulse is stated as so many beats a minute.
c. Count the beats for half a minute, and multiply by 2.

The resting heart rate shows considerable variation ranging between 50 and 120 beats per minute (BPM).

a. The parasympathetic and sympathetic components of the autonomic nervous system have a major effect on heart rate.
b. Tachycardia HR > 100 BPM.
   Causes
   i. Exercise
   ii. Fever
   iii. Thyrotoxicosis
c. Bradycardia HR < 50 BPM.
   Causes
   iv. Athletes
   v. Myxoedema

2. *Rhythm*
Decide whether the rhythm is:
a. Regular. Sinus arrhythmia is the normal variation with respiration. The rate slows with inspiration and quickens with expiration as the intrathoracic pressure alters the venous return and cardiac output.
b. Regularly irregular.
   Causes
   i. Pulses bigeminous
   ii. Coupled extrasystole.
c. Irregularly irregular.
   Causes
   iii. AF
   iv. Multiple extrasystoles.

Character of the vessel wall
Arteriosclerosis is indicated by rings felt in the wall or by a stiff and tortuous vessel.

3. Character of the abnormal pulse.
It is not usually possible to detect slight variations from the normal but in certain diseases the character of the pulse is detectably abnormal.

It is best felt by palpating the carotid artery, at the level of thyroid cartilage.

The most important abnormal forms of the arterial pulse wave are:

a. Anacrotic or slow rising pulse.
It is of small volume with a late systolic peak.
Cause: aortic stenosis.

b. Collapsing or Water hammer pulse.
It is characterised by a rapid upstroke and rapid descent of the pulse wave. Best felt with the palm of the hand against the patient's forearm held above the level of the heart.

A prerequisite for the production of collapsing pulse is a wide pulse pressure which can by caused by three groups of conditions.

A. Rapid run off of blood from the arterial system.
  i.   Central causes
      - Aortic regurgitation (commonest cause)
      - Severe Mitral Regurgitation
      - Rupture of sinus of Valsalva
      - Large Ventral Septal Defect
      - Large Patent Ductus Arteriosis
  ii. Peripheral causes
      - Arterial-venous fistula
      - Multiple small arterial-venous fistula
      - Paget's disease
      - Hepatic failure

B. Complete heart block

C. Hyperkinetic circulation with peripheral vasodilation
      - Pregnancy
      - Anxiety
      - Fever
      - Thyrotoxicosis
      - Severe anaemia
      - Exercise
      - Hypercarbia
      - Beri-Beri.

c. Pulses paradoxus:
Paradox: the heart sounds may be still heard over the precordium when no pulse is palpable at radial artery.

It is an exaggeration of the normal response to respiration of a change in blood pressure of 5–10 mmHg. An increase in the variation in blood pressure by more than 10–12 mmHg between inspiration and expiration occurs with:
  - Pericardial tamponade
  - Constrictive pericarditis
  - Restrictive cardiomyopathy
  - Asthma exacerbation
  - COAD exacerbation
  - PE
  - Pregnancy.

d. Pulsus alternans. Alternating weak and strong pulse beats.
Causes
- Severe congestive heart failure
- Any cause of a rapid respiratory rate.

e. Bisferiens pulse. A pulse wave form with two up strokes.
Causes
- Exercise
- Fever
- Patent Ductus Arteriosus
- Double aorta.

Volume

This gives a rough guide to the pulse pressure, which depends on:

- Stroke volume
- Compliance of the arteries.

Is best assessed in the carotid and brachial artery because they are less likely to be modified by alterations in the properties of the peripheral vessel.

The pulse pressure = Systolic BP – Diastolic BP.

Causes of a wide or increase in pulse pressure:

- Aortic Regurgitation
- Patent Ductus Arteriosus
- Sinus bradycardia
- Fever
- Anaemia
- Strenuous exercise
- Thyrotoxicosis.

Causes of a narrow pulse pressure:

- Congestive Cardiac Failure
- Aortic Stenosis
- Dehydration
- Severe Mitral Regurgitation
- Atherosclerosis.

Synchronicity

Check if there is a synchronicity between the right and the left radial pulses.

Causes of lack of synchronicity

- Congenital anomaly
- Dissecting aneurysm
- Previous catheterisation.

Delay

Delay of the femoral compared with the right radial pulse is found in coarctation of aorta.

Answers – Self-test: Taking the pulse

1. Rate, rhythm – regular or irregular, volume, the nature of the pulse and the artery wall. You should count the pulse for a full minute if possible or explain that you are doing it for 30 seconds. Feel both radial arteries and the femoral arteries.

   Atherosclerotic rings may be felt in the arterial wall.

   Small volume pulse pressure: aortic stenosis, low blood pressure or low cardiac output.

2. Collapsing: raise arm above heart to feel the column of blood as if it were transiently banging against the palpating fingers (also called a water hammer pulse).

3. Present with aortic incompetence, hyperdynamic circulation as in thyrotoxicosis, AV fistulae.

4. Allen's test. Identify radial and ulnar arteries at wrist. Squeeze hand to exsanguinate it. Occlude radial and ulnar arteries – check by seeing pale hand.

   Release ulnar artery and watch re-perfusion of hand indicating perfusion through a patent ulnar artery and palmar arch vessels in hand.

5. Positive test – no ulnar flow.

6. Allen was originally interested in diagnosing endarteritis obliterans of the digital arteries.

7. Pulsus alternans is alternating strong and weak beats seen in left ventricular failure.

8. The pulse volume normally increases in inspiration due to a reduced intrathoracic pressure and an increased venous return to the heart; this will give a reduction in heart rate in young fit patients – sinus arrhythmia. The change of heart rate with respiration – beat to beat variation is a sign of competent cardiovascular reflexes and disappears in disease and anaesthesia.

   Pulsus paradoxus. Normally blood pressure changes by 5–10 mmHg during the respiratory cycle. An increase in this variation in blood pressure occurs in: pericardial effusion and constrictive pericarditis, severe asthma, and gives a pulsus paradoxus.

9. Arterial catheterisation may be complicated by: infection, haemorrhage, arteriovenous fistula, complete occlusion of the artery leading to finger ischaemia and gangrene, embolisation to the finger(s), the injection of incompatible materials.

Answers – Physical examination 4

1. *a.* *Inspect* the neck for pulsation deep to Sternomastoid.

    Compress the liver in the abdomen. The venous pressure should rise confirming the internal jugular vein (hepato-jugular reflex).

    Look for the uppermost point of distension of the right internal jugular vein.
   b. *Measure* the vertical height of the internal jugular venous pulse above the manubrio-sternal angle.
   c. *Identify the waves* in neck vein
      a wave – produced by right atrial contraction. Before the carotid pulse.
      c wave – close of the tricuspid valve. Bulging of the tricuspid valve into the right atrium as the ventricle contracts against a closed pulmonary valve.
      v wave – rises with filling of the right atrium.
      x descent between a and c waves. During relaxation of the atrium.
      y descent between c and v waves. During atrial emptying.

2. a wave absent in:

    ▪ AF due to poor/no atrial contraction.

    Large when atrial pressure is high:

    ▪ in tricuspid and pulmonary stenosis, right ventricular hypertrophy, atrial septal defect, pulmonary hypertension.

    Cannon waves are present in complete heart block.
    v wave large in tricuspid incompetence.
    x descent absent in tricuspid incompetence.
    y descent steep in right ventricular failure, and constrictive pericarditis.

3. Venous pulsation:

    ▪ Cannot be palpated.
    ▪ Can be abolished by gentle digital pressure.
    ▪ Varies with posture and respiration. Falls in inspiration.
    ▪ Is raised by abdominal pressure and Valsalva manoeuvre.
    ▪ May cause pulsation in the ear lobe when very high.
    ▪ Two waves in venous pulse to one in arterial pulse.

4. ▪ Low CVP, low systolic pressure = Hypovolaemia. Treatment fluid loading.
    ▪ Normal CVP, low systolic pressure = peripheral circulatory failure. Treatment inotrope, vasoconstrictor.
    ▪ High CVP, low BP = CHF, constrictive pericarditis, cardiac tamponade.

    The CVP, by itself, only records the right heart filling pressure = pre-load (not cardiac function).

Answers – Physical examination 5

1. Practise taking the blood pressure with a mercury sphygmomanometer. You may not have done it for some time. The patient should be positioned so that the arm, cuff and sphygmomanometer are all at the same level as the heart.

2. Measure the pressure in both arms. There may be coarctation of the aorta or an AV fistula.

3. Korotkoff.

4. First sound.

5. Fifth sound. Except in hyperdynamic states such as seen in pregnancy when the fourth sound is usually taken as the diastolic pressure.

6. Medial to and under the medial border of biceps; medial to the biceps tendon.

7. Cuff bladder length = Twice the width.
   Width of the cuff should be the diameter of arm + 20%, or half of the circumference (circumference is about 3 times the diameter (22/7)).

8. It will over read the pressure.

9. The systolic pressure reading will be higher in the foot than if read in the aorta or brachial artery.

Indirect blood pressure measurement
Introduce yourself and explain procedure.

Use a sequence:

- The patient should be relaxed and lying supine.
- Start by feeling the pulses in all four limbs.
- Use the right arm, unless not available. The arm pressures should be within 10 mmHg of each other, but rarely the same.
- Choose the correct size cuff. The width should be 20% greater than the diameter. A small cuff will act as a tourniquet and cause over-reading.
- The bladder of the cuff should be centred over the brachial artery.
- The cuff is inflated up to 50% above systolic pressure. At this stage the systolic pressure is estimated by palpation – feeling when the pulse is lost as the cuff is inflated.
- The cuff pressure is now deflated until the Korotkoff sounds are heard. These sounds are due to turbulent flow under the cuff.

The mercury sphygmomanometer must read zero at the start. It must be used vertical and kept at the same level as the arm. Other devices are calibrated using a mercury column with a filter in the line.

Automatic devices inflate the cuff and then slowly reduce the pressure at 2–3 mmHg/second. A cuff that over inflates too often and only slowly deflates can cause trauma to the arm tissues and nerves.

The Korotkoff Sounds

1. First appearance systolic pressure
2. Reduced sound
3. Increased sound
4. Reduced sound
5. Loss of sound taken as diastolic expect when the circulation is hyperdynamic and the sounds continue then 4 is taken.

Answers – Self-test: Blood pressure measurement

1. There is a slight reduction in systolic pressure <20 mmHg and a rise in diastolic pressure <10 mmHg

2. The systolic and diastolic pressure fall on standing.

3. It is a **D**evice for **I**ndirect **N**on-invasive **A**utomated **M**ean **A**rterial **P**ressure measurement.

4. It is a microprocessor, which controls the sequence of inflation and deflation. The cuff is inflated to systolic pressure + 30 mmHg. Then deflated at 2–3 mmHg/second.

   The blood flowing under the cuff causes turbulence and oscillations. The transducer senses the amount of turbulence.

5. Systolic – Onset of rapid oscillations.
   Diastolic – Onset of decreasing oscillation.
   Mean – maximum oscillation at lowest cuff pressure.

6. Absolute values: water column for CVP, mercury sphygmomanometer for BP. Calibration: Pulse oximeter, Pressure transducer, Capnograph, Oxygen analyser.

7. Ideally three reference points are used. In some cases only two are easily available.
   a. Oxygen analysers: Use 21% Air and 100% oxygen.
   b. Capnograph. Use air 0% and a known concentration from a cylinder.
   c. Pulse oximeter. Use zero open to the air and a group of healthy volunteers to give 100%.
   d. Direct pressure. Connect transducer to a saline-filled manometer tube, a three-way tap, a filter to a mercury sphygmomanometer. Open the tap to air gives zero. Fill a syringe with saline. Attach a syringe to the port open to air and turn tap so that a syringe can pressurise both the transducer and the mercury column.

      Increase pressure to 100 mmHg on column and calibrate traducer at this level. A third point may be taken at 200 mmHg.

8. *Drift* is the tendency for the reading to vary from the actual value. The difference of the reading from the actual value becomes more marked the further away from the calibration points.

   Gain is amplification. The scale for the reading may be increased. Any increase in scale will tend to increase any difference from the actual reading.

Answers – Physical examination 6

1. The praecordium is the term used to indicate the anterior aspect of the chest, which overlies the heart.

2. Introduce yourself.
   - Ask permission to examine the patient.

3. You should always use the same routine.
   - Inspection
   - Palpation
   - Percussion
   - Auscultation.

Guidance

1. Inspection
   Inspect the praecordium for:
   a. Chest deformities such as
      - Kyphosis, scoliosis, barrel chest which may cause heart failure.
      - Funnel chest may be a part of Marfan's syndrome.
      - Any prominence of the chest wall.
   b. Pulsations
      - Forceful apical impulse in left ventricular hypertrophy.
      - Pulsation in the second left intercostal space – due to enlarged pulmonary artery.
      - Pulsation in the second right intercostal space or upper sternum due to an aortic aorta.
      - Whole chest may move when there is severe cardiomegaly.
      Epigastric pulsation. Consider:
         - Aortic pulsation in asthenic people
         - Overlying tumour
         - Right ventricular hypertrophy
         - Tricuspid regurge
         - Aneurysm of aorta.

2. Palpation
   - The patient should be in recumbent position.
   - The intercostal spaces are localised with reference to the sternal angle of Louis, which corresponds to the lower border of the second rib.
   a. Palpate for:
      - Apex beat:
        This is the furthest point away from the mid line and the furthest point downwards where a cardiac pulsation can be felt.
        Normally is situated in the fifth intercostal space 1 cm internal to the mid clavicular line. It can be felt more easily if the patient lies on their left side.
   b. Character
      i. Displaced. The apex beat is displaced outwards and downwards by

left ventricular hypertrophy. Associated with high BP, aortic valve disease (AS, AI), mitral incompetence and VSD.

ii. Heave. Right ventricular hypertrophy shifts the apex out but there is a greater pulse to the left of the sternum, which gives a heaving, or lifting. (The right ventricle is behind and to the left of the sternum; the left ventricle is behind the right ventricle until it becomes anterior laterally).

iii. Tapping. Is a palpable first sound, usually of mitral stenosis. It occurs due to the sharp closure of the mitral valve (sensation of hard knock on other side of closed door).

iv. Diffuse impulse. The apex beat is not the most prominent sensation in right ventricular hypertrophy.

c. Displaced apex beat
Causes
   i. Cardiac
      - Congenital – dextrocardia
      - Acquired:
        - LVH – shifted down and out
        - RVH – shifted out
   ii. Pulmonary
      - Pushed:
        - Pleural effusion
        - Pneumothorax
      - Pulled:
        - Pulmonary fibrosis
        - Collapse
      - Deformity of thoracic cage
        - Scoliosis
        - Kyphoscohiosis.

d. Impalpable apex beat.
Causes
   i. Physiological
      - Thick chest.wall
      - Lying behind the rib
      - Large breast in females
   ii. Pathological
      - Pericardial effusion
      - Emphysema
      - Dextrocardia.

e. Thrill is a palpable murmur.
Causes
   - Systolic thrill at the apex. Mitral incompetence
   - Diastolic thrill at the apex. Mitral stenosis
   - Systolic thrill at the lower left sternal edge. Ventricular septal defect
   - Systolic thrill at the upper left sternal edge. Aortic stenosis, pulmonary stenosis.

f. **Parasternal heave**
Palpate firmly the left border of the sternum.
A heave suggests right ventricular hypertrophy = dominant right heart.

g. **Other palpable sounds**
- Palpable first heart sound in Mitral Stenosis
- Palpable second heart sound
  - In pulmonary area – pulmonary hypertension
  - In aortic area – systemic hypertension
- Palpable third and fourth heart sounds

Any other pulsations
Any tenderness over the chest.

3. **Percussion**
Percussion of the heart is now seldom carried out as it adds little to the clinical assessment.

4. **Auscultation**
- Heart sounds
- Added sounds
- Murmurs.

Heart murmurs are due to turbulent blood flow. A systolic murmur occurs between the first and second sound and coincides with the apex beat.

Systolic murmurs occur when blood passes through a part open aortic or pulmonary stenosis or part closed mitral or tricuspid incompetence.

Diastolic murmurs occur when blood is flowing through part closed aortic or pulmonary incompetence or a part open mitral of tricuspid stenosis.

A VSD causes a systolic murmur, an ASD causes a murmur due to excess blood flowing through the pulmonary valve. A patent ductus causes a continuous machinery murmur.

Incompetence murmurs extend throughout systole but decrease through diastole.

Mitral murmurs are best heard at the apex, tricuspid murmurs at the lower left sternal edge, pulmonary murmurs at the upper left sternal edge and aortic murmurs along the left sternal edge.

Answers – Self-test: Cardiovascular system

1. Finger clubbing can be caused by cyanotic heart disease and infective endocarditis. Other causes include chronic suppurative lung diseases, chronic lower bowel conditions and, cancer of the lung.

   Splinter haemorrhages are seen in trauma, embolisation and subacute endocarditis.

2. Pulse for rate, rhythm, volume nature e.g. collapsing and character of wall.

3. Blood pressure – if hypertensive consider examining the fundus of the eye and other limbs for evidence of coarctation.

4. Cyanosis is a bluish discolouration of the lips, mucous membranes and tongue. This indicates that more than 5 g/100ml of haemoglobin is desaturated.

5. Face. Cyanosis, malar flush.

6. *a.* The venous pulse is seen but not felt; has a double wave, is increased in height by a Valsalva manoeuvre and pressure on the liver. The height of the venous pulse wave will alter with posture and goes down with inspiration.
   b. Landmarks for the internal jugular pulse. Deep to sternomastoid. The internal jugular vein runs from the angle of the mandible to a point behind the clavicle about 2 fingers width from the mid-line. The vertical height of filling in the vein above the manubrium-sternal angle may give a measure of the pressure in the right atrium.
   c. The normal venous wave is an "a" wave coinciding with atrial contraction, a "c" wave transmitted from the carotid artery, a "v" wave due to pressure of atrial filling while the tricuspid valve is closed.
   d. Tricuspid incompetence will give a larger "v" wave.
   e. Ask the patient to do a Valsalva manoeuvre to distend the veins, or gently palpate and put pressure on the liver. Ask if the liver is tender first.

7. Oedema occurs when the capillary pressure exceeds the oncotic pressure. A raised right atrial pressure leading to a raised venous pressure will lead to symmetrical peripheral oedema. Venous or lymphatic obstruction will give an asymmetrical oedema. You should know Starling's equation.

8. The apex beat is the furthest point outward and downwards that a cardiac impulse can be felt. It is normally in the mid clavicular line and 5th intercostal space but it will be further out with left ventricular enlargement. Right heart enlargement will cause a lifting to the left of the sternum detected by the flat of the hand.

9. Auscultation may be used to detect the nature of the first and second sounds as the flow through the valves suddenly changes. Murmurs are due to turbulent flow through a valve. A systolic murmur occurs when the

mitral and tricuspid valves should be shut. The commonest cause in the elderly is noise of flow through an arteriosclerotic aorta. It may be back flow through an incompetent mitral or tricuspid valve or a ventricular septal defect or forward flow through a stenosed aortic or pulmonary valve. The murmur of an ASD is the excessive flow of blood through a normal pulmonary valve. Diastolic murmurs occur when the mitral and tricuspid valves are open and the aortic and pulmonary valves closed. Mitral diastolic murmurs are difficult to hear but there are clues that they will be present. The clues are: a history of rheumatic heart disease; the presence of a mitral systolic murmur as stenosis and incompetence often go together; the opening snap after the second sound in diastole and just before the diastolic murmur.

Answers – Self-test 1: Cranial nerves

1. Test for smell: The response to smell is variable. The test requires specific materials which are unlikely to be available other than in neurological clinics. So this nerve will usually be passed over unless proper samples are available. You might ask about head injury, obvious anosmia or a related change in taste. Otherwise miss this cranial nerve.

2. Test for:
   a. Fundus and visual acuity.
   b. Pupil size and pupillary reflexes.
   c. Visual fields.

   Examine the fundus, particularly for changes associated with hypertension and diabetes. Test for blindness by asking the patient to read a few words.

   Test fields of vision for temporal and nasal loss. Temporal loss occurs with pituitary tumours – can you explain how? Variable field losses with multiple sclerosis.

   Look at the symmetry of the sizes of the pupils. Exclude Horner's syndrome.

   Reflexes – involving cranial nerves 2 and 3. The pupil should constrict when a light is brought in from the side – indicating a light reflex. The opposite pupil should also constrict indicating a consensual light reflex. Test accommodation by moving an object, such as your finger, in towards the eye from a distance away. The pupil should constrict.

3. Test for: Eye movement – eye and eyelid movement and sympathetic eye innervation.

   Third: Innervates most of the extrinsic eye muscles moving the eye upwards and medially. It also raises the upper lid.

   The fourth (trochlear) is limited to the superior oblique muscle rotating the eye down.

   Sixth (abducent) to the lateral rectus muscle, moves the eye laterally.

   In a third nerve palsy the eye is down and out.

   A ptosis may be unilateral due to:

   ▪ A third nerve palsy with a dilated pupil and eye movement limited to "down and out".
   ▪ A Horner's syndrome with a small pupil.
   ▪ A lower motor seventh palsy (see under 5)

   or bilateral due to:

   ▪ Myasthenia gravis.
   ▪ Myotonia dystrophica

   Nystagmus involves several nerve pathways. It consists of a slow movement in one direction and a fast movement back. Its presence may indicate a defect in the cerebellum, brain stem or less commonly the cerebral hemispheres.

Brain death tests involve testing for nystagmus by putting cold water into the ear to test the vestibular nerve. A normal response is a slow movement towards and fast away from the cold stimulus.

4. Test:
   - Sensation of the face.
   - Three divisions

   Ophthalmic: Forehead including tip of nose – also the cornea.
   Maxillary: Cheek from lower eyelid to upper lip including side of nose and palate.
   Mandibular: Lower lip and chin.
   Test with light touch – cotton wool on cornea and skin, then pin prick to skin.
   Also taste to anterior two-thirds of tongue from the seventh via the chorda tympani.

   Motor fibres to muscles of mastication, particularly masseter. Ask to grin, look for a hollow in the temporal fossa and test by opening the mouth against a resistance. Try biting on a spatula.

5. Test: Motor power to facial muscles: Ask to grimace by screwing up face, eyes tight closed, raise forehead.

   Consider the following situations. Distinguish weakness due to an upper motor neurone (UMN) deficit, e.g. a CVA; from a lower motor neurone (LMN) weakness of Bell's palsy (a virus infection affecting the facial nerve in the ear). In a LMN lesion the mouth is pulled to the opposite side by a smile and the eye rolls up under the eyelid rather than the eyelid closing tightly on the affected side. The lower neurone lesion affects all of the side of the face including one side of the forehead. In an UMN lesion the forehead muscles contract on both sides, the eyes close and the blinking is preserved due to bilateral upper motor neurone control. Nerve damage due to a parotid lesion or during parotid surgery will give variable weaknesses. If a ptosis is bilateral consider myasthenia gravis.

6. Test: Hearing by talking into ear or a tuning fork held near to the ear. This also tests the ossicle system in the middle ear. Tuning fork to the mastoid bone tests for a conduction deafness.

   Weber's test distinguishes conduction from nerve deafness. A high pitch tuning fork is plucked and then placed against the middle of the forehead. The sound is heard best in the normal ear if nerve deafness, or best in deaf ear if conduction deafness. If heard equally no deafness, or ears are equally deaf.

7. Test: Taste to the posterior one third of tongue and by eliciting the gag reflex. Test for difficulty in swallowing.

8. The vagus, or wanderer, innervates the thoracic and abdominal viscera.

Test: The recurrent laryngeal nerve is best tested by observing the movement of the cords at laryngoscopy. Weakness may cause hoarseness or an impaired force to coughing. A nerve weakness may occur at thyroid surgery and with lesions at the apex of the lung.

9. Test: Motor function of sternomastoid and trapezius.

Trapezius. Shrug shoulders. Sternomastoid turn head to one side against resistance.

10. Motor innervation to tongue.

Test: Protrude tongue straight out.

Answers – Self-Test 2: Cranial nerves

1. The eye is affected in a number of ways:

   - Cataracts
   - Retinal haemorrhages and exudates
   - Reduced vision due to macular damage
   - Retinal ischaemia and new vessel formation.

2. In the mid line pressing on the centre of the optic chiasma, probably due to a lesion of the pituitary gland, craniopharyngioma, or secondary tumour.

3. Miosis, enophthalmos, ptosis, anhydrosis (plus nasal stuffiness not classically described by Horner). The conjunctival blood vessels may be dilated. All due to a lesion of sympathetic innervation to the head.

4. Lesion of

   - Sympathetic innervation, Horner's syndrome,
   - Third, or
   - Seventh cranial nerve palsy, probably lower motor neurone e.g. Bell's palsy.

5. Fifth cranial nerve and masseter muscle.

6. Seventh cranial nerve via the chorda tympani to the peripheral part of the fifth cranial nerve.

7. A conduction deafness in the right ear.

8. Ask the patient to swallow. Gag reflex elicited if an object is placed towards the back of the mouth or tongue.

9. Hoarseness or a poor force of cough.

10. Trapezius – shrugging of the shoulders. Sternomastoid – rotating the head against a resistance.

Answers – Self-test 1: CNS

1. Ask the patient to walk a short distance and observe the gait which may indicate: a hemiplegia, stiff and jerky due to spasticity.
   Parkinsonism – small shuffling steps, difficult to start and stop walking, everything appears stiff.
   Test: Stand patient upright with eyes closed. Ask patient to hold hand out level with the face, point the index finger and then bring it to the nose. If the patient fails to bring the finger directly to the nose there is a cerebellar disorder; but exclude a deficit in joint position sense or a motor weakness.
   Cerebellar disease may be associated with a terminal intention tremor.
   Test: For coordination of upper limb by finger – nose pointing.
   Lower limb by heel – shin slide.
   Rapid, repetitive movement of the hands for disdiadokokinesis.

2. Test motor function
   ▪ Look at the position of the limb for an obvious palsy; then look at the muscles for wasting and fasciculations.
   ▪ Palpate the muscle tone which can be flaccid with a lower motor neurone lesion. Increased tone can be either clasp knife: that is stiff to start with and then gives way in cerebral lesions like a CVA, or cogwheel: that is stiff throughout as in Parkinsonism with a pill rolling tremor which stops when doing something.
   ▪ Reflexes
   Test the nerve arc from stretch receptors to spinal cord and back to muscle.

   Upper limb: Biceps (C5, 6), Triceps (C7, 8), Brachio radialis (C5, 6).
   Lower limb: Knee (L4) and Ankle (S1). Dorsiflexion of the hallux depends on L5.

   Know the dermatomes of each reflex tested. An absent ankle reflex may not be significant in the elderly.

   Plantar reflex. The stimulus should be applied along the lateral border of the foot.

   In the presence of an upper motor neurone lesion, such as in the pyramidal tracts, the big toe extends. Stimulating the sole of the foot will produce a withdrawal reflex.

3. Tests of sensory function
   ▪ Light touch and vibration pass in the dorsal columns on the same side of the spinal cord, only crossing to the other side in the medulla.
   ▪ Pain with temperature pass to the contralateral anterior lateral spinothalamic tracts.

   Test with cotton wool for light touch and a tuning fork on bony promontories for vibration sense. Test for pain and cold with a pin and an alcohol wipe. Test on the trunk for a sensory level with a cold alcohol wipe.

Typically, in syringomyelia, pain is lost on one side and light touch on the other.

Test both pain and light touch for loss of dermatome innervation and for specific nerve distribution. For instance: an ulnar nerve palsy will give loss of sensation to the palm and dorsum of the hand affecting the little finger and the ulnar half of the ring finger. In a C8 dermatome lesion, the sensory loss will extend up the forearm to the antecubital fossa on the ulnar side.

4. The patient lies supine.
   Straight leg raising. Passively raise the ankle with the knee extended. This tests limitation of sciatic nerve root mobility and posterior lumbar muscle tone. Pain before 90° arises due to sciatic nerve root tethering, pressure, or posterior lumbar muscle spasm.

   Sciatic stretch. Lift the ankle and flex the knee and hip. Ensure there is no pain due to knee or hip disease. Pain is due to sciatic nerve or muscle spasm as with SLR.

   The patient lies prone.

   Femoral stretch. The ankle is lifted and the knee is flexed with the hip extended. Exclude knee or hip disease. Pain is due to femoral nerve root irritation or anterior muscle spasm (psoas and iliacus).

Answers – Self-Test 2: CNS

1. Upper trunk paralysis C5 affects the muscles: deltoid, biceps, brachioradialis and brachialis. The arm hangs down by the side, medially rotated, forearm extended and pronated. Shoulder abduction and elbow flexion is lost. This is Erb's palsy or waiters tip position.

   A lower trunk C8, T1 paralysis affects the small muscles of the hand and flexion of the wrist and fingers is lost. The unchecked extension gives a claw hand or Klumpke's palsy.

2. C7 and 8.

3. *a.* Radial nerve lesion.
   - Motor loss leads to lack of hand extension and so a dropped wrist.
   - Sensory loss on the dorsum of the hand on the radial side.
   b. Median nerve lesion.
   - Motor loss produces an ape like hand with lack of thenar muscle action and flexion of the hand may be weak.
   - Sensory loss of palmar surface of hand and fingers except for the little finger and part of the ring finger.
   c. Ulnar nerve lesion.
   - Motor loss is an inability to stretch out the fingers and hypothenar wasting.
   - The hand appears clawed.
   - Sensory loss over the ulnar side of the hand on palmar and dorsal surfaces.

4. T2.

5. T10.

6. L5.

7. The skin over the medial calf is supplied by the saphenous nerve, a branch of the femoral nerve. Dermatome L4.

8. Idiopathic loss of dopamine neurotransmitter in the substantia nigra, post-encephalitic, drug-induced, e.g. phenothiazines – particularly piperazines, butyrophenones.

9. Drugs: Dopaminergic, e.g. L-dopa with a dopa-decarboxylase inhibitor (carbidopa or benserazide) to reduce L-dopa metabolism. A monoamine oxidase B inhibitor – selegiline. Antimuscarinic – orphenadrine or benzhexol. Muscle relaxant and anti-tremor drugs, e.g. diazepam.

10. Damage to the nerve root of L4; multiple sclerosis; causes of myopathies, e.g. inflammation, alcohol, hypokalaemia; causes of peripheral neuropathies, diabetes, malignancy, Guillain-Barré syndrome, toxicity: regional anaesthesia and during recovery from general anaesthesia.

Answers – Physical examination 9

1. Airway
Stabilise the neck until it is proven that it is not broken.

Open mouth, sweep finger round inside to remove loose teeth, detect vomit and blood.

Breathing: inspect for evidence of breathing. Feel warm air with palm of hand against open mouth. Hear respiratory sounds, see rise and fall of abdomen with diaphragmatic movement. Check that the chest moves at the same time and not paradoxically indicating obstruction.

Circulation feel pulse at radial, carotid and on both sides.

2. Glasgow Coma Scale
- Eye opening:
  - 4 – Eyes wide open
  - 3 – Eyes open to command
  - 2 – Eyes open to pain
  - 1 – Shut
- Response to command
  - 5 – Orientated
  - 4 – Confused sentences
  - 3 – Confused words
  - 2 – Noises
  - 1 – None
- Motor response
  - 6 – Moves limbs to command
  - 5 – Localises to pain
  - 4 – Withdraws to pain
  - 3 – Abnormal flexion
  - 2 – Extension
  - 1 – None

Maximum score 15, less than 9 consider intubation to protect airway and ensure oxygenation.

Pupil size. A unilateral, dilated pupil suggests an intracranial haematoma on that side. Bilaterally, constricted pupils suggest either the effect of an opioid or brain stem damage.

Limb tone and sensation. Loss of tone, power or sensation on one side suggest a unilateral haematoma on that side. An extensor reflex suggests brain stem damage.

Answers – Physical examination 10

1. Introduce yourself

General examination
- Weight, nutritional status, build.
- Hydration, particularly if nausea and vomiting or urinary frequency.
- Colour of skin may be hyperpigmented, spider naevi due to oestrogen, palmar erythema – but exclude liver disease. Look at the conjunctiva or mucous membranes for anaemia, perfusion, and jaundice.
- Temperature.

CVS
- Pulse rate – high, rhythm – normal, volume – collapsing. All compatible with high cardiac output.
- Apex beat will be displace up and out (left axis deviation) due to pressure on the diaphragm.
- JVP and pulsations. Venous access.
- BP may be raised in pre-eclampsia, systolic murmur due to increased flow through pulmonary or tricuspid valves.
- Important pathological murmurs are pan or late systolic, or vary with respiration.
- Sacral and ankle oedema.

Respiration
- Breathlessness.

Abdomen
- Assess fundal height: 12 weeks above symphysis pubis, 20 weeks at umbilicus.
- Constipation may be evident.
- Abdominal scars.

CNS
- Cranial and peripheral nerves, particularly if considering a regional block.
- Fundi exclude papilloedema.

Musculoskeletal
- Spine for deformity, infection, palpate spaces. If considering an epidural.

Renal
- Test urine for glucose and protein.

COMMUNICATION

3

Introduction

Doctors find themselves in difficulty because of poor communication skills. The patient feels they were not fully informed, an issue has not been made clear, or no apology was given when there was an error or a mistake.

Good communication requires various skills including:

- Listening skills. An ability to hear what the patient is trying to express and not to impose a stereotype response.
- Knowledge and the ability to explain clearly, in words that are understandable.
- The ability to organise thoughts and ideas into a logical order.
- Honesty, to tell the truth with kindness but not to avoid the truth, even to the point that the patient or relative is frightened to proceed or becomes emotionally upset.
- Tact, compassion, sympathy (the ability to feel sorry for the patient) and empathy (the ability to understand how the patient feels) to help a distressed patient.
- Patience and the ability to try to understand another person's point of view.
- In medicine, it is better to request than demand.
- Time. Good communication cannot be rushed. Offer to return again.

It is important to understand how we communicate and what makes for good communication.

- Verbal communication is what we say.
- Body language is the way in which we use our body gestures to express ourselves.

It is suggested that up to 80% of all communication is non-verbal.

The way in which we use our eyes, facial expression and posture, all impart meaning.

There are various forms of communication and, in an examination, there will be examples of some of these: explanation, reassurance, negotiation, expression of an opinion or judgement (forms of communication that are unlikely to be in an examination are a social chat, lecture or command).

When all is well, communication is not difficult. When there is a problem, then various aspects of communication can become a problem.

The process of good communication

Establish a relationship
Introduce yourself and identify who you are. Establish who is the patient or other person to whom you are speaking. Avoid mistakes in identity.

Appearance
Clothing, punctuality, not fidgeting and eye contact are likely to mean that more confidence and attention is given to what is being said.

Dress should be appropriate to age, especially children. Avoid giving the impression of being hurried. Meeting patients in theatre clothes will impart a sense of not having time and discourages a full discussion with time for questions. In the examination, dress should be comfortable, bearing in mind that there is a lot of moving around to be accomplished, work on manikins and a resuscitation station.

Identify the problem
What is the patient worried about, what has gone wrong, what needs to be explained? Do not impose your own ideas. Be precise about the problem. If there is a protocol or guidelines, use them. What is the situation? Or what request is being made? Then prepare for the follow-up and related questions.

Give the correct information
Where knowledge is required it must be accurate. If you do not know the answer, say so and seek advice from other doctors or books. Be truthful, do not give hope if there is none. Give options and alternatives if there are any. Use words that are understandable to the patient. Do not miss anything out because it is difficult, upsetting or rare. It is increasingly important that patients and relatives are told everything. Informed consent requires that all the common problems are discussed that could happen in 1 in 100 or more cases, and all other serious problems. This virtually means, discuss everything.

How would you want your family to be treated?
In practice the *my child test* is a good way to assess the appropriateness of the information and approach. If you would do this for your child then it is probably good. If you have reservations about this advice/treatment for your child then think about what needs to be changed.

Principles of good communication that are often missed out
- Introduce yourself.
- Find out what the patient is worried about and allow the patient to express their problem.
- Admit your own limitations.
- Say sorry if there has been an error or a less than satisfactory outcome.
- If you do not know, say so and that you will find out or seek a second opinion.
- Do not try to blame.
- The patient is entitled to know everything but some patients do not want to know everything. Try to satisfy the patient's needs.

- If a person is difficult or cross, still be polite, do not lose your temper.
- Be polite but clear about the problem. Take your time. Do not be rushed.
- When dealing with difficult staff, be polite but clear about your needs. Make reasonable demands; compromise if possible but if patient safety is at risk say so.
- Do not use threats.
- When offering an explanation use facts not opinions.
- Try to explain matters as simply as possible. If it is a patient, use words they will understand; ask, "Do you understand?" If talking to another colleague, use medical terms.
- Check that all has been understood. Offer to come back and follow-up.
- Do not trivialise something if the patient thinks it is important.
- Tell the truth with kindness, do not lie or mislead.
- Be responsive to other people's problems.
- Say "Please" and "Thank you".
- Keep a written record of anything that may be controversial. If in doubt, get written consent. Give the patient/relative a copy of written details. If in doubt, have a chaparone or a witness.

Examples of communication situations
- Explain a procedure.
- Comfort/reassure a person who is distressed.
- Obtain consent.
- Deal with a difficult situation.
- Explain a complication.
- Deal with staff.

Communication 1

(Answers on page 111)

You are to see the wife of a patient. Her husband was admitted 6 hours ago following a massive cerebral haemorrhage confirmed by brain scan and his lungs are being ventilated.

Use the 90 seconds in the waiting period to mentally rehearse some of the issues involved.

Introduce yourself.

In real life it is important to check that you are speaking to the right person, before discussing confidential information.

Establish the background. You may be in a hurry but allow time to find out about the situation from the patient's point of view.

"Tell me what you know of what has happened" or "What have you been told so far?"

The woman says that she knows her husband has no hope of recovery.

Questions

1. Write down the first point(s) that you think is(are) relevant and how you will deal with it(them).

2. What are the main issues that you will cover?

   The woman wants assurance that her husband is dead.

3. What will you say?

   She has accepted your explanation. Move to the next issue.

4. What has to be discussed after brain death tests?

   In these circumstances it may be necessary to consult the coroner.

5. What will you say about the coroner?

   Finish by offering sympathy and express sadness at what has happened.

Communication 2 (Answers on page 112)

You are to see a mother who is anxious about her son. The son is to have an anaesthetic for insertions of grommets.

This as an exercise in four parts.
- Find out what has to be explained. In this case what is the cause of the anxiety.
- Find out why it is a problem and what is already known or understood.
- Give a clear explanation to relieve the anxiety.
- Check that there are no other problems and that the explanation has been accepted. Do not go into the situation with any preconceived ideas. This means do not explain something that the patient is not concerned about and miss their problem in the process.

Take the 90 seconds between stations to consider what issues might be causes for anxiety.

Questions

1. List the possible reasons for anxiety.

Introduction – You should say who you are, ask their name.

Rapport and a little background information. Establish a rapport by checking the name and age of the child. Then go straight to the point. "Tell me about your anxiety", or "What are you most concerned about?"

Ask open-ended questions. That is, questions that cannot easily be answered by a "Yes" or "No" reply. Allow the person to tell you, preferably without interruption, about their problem.

The mother is concerned because her nephew did not recover from an operation 6 years ago.

2. At this point, formulate a list of possible explanations.

You may need to clarify whether he died or if recovery was delayed?

"Tell me more about your nephew." "What do you mean by saying he did not recover?" The nephew had a tonsillectomy but did not breathe properly after surgery. In recovery he was ventilated for 3 hours before waking up. You may have to clarify with the mother that it was due to the muscle relaxant.

You are now expected to explain suxamethonium apnoea to this mother.

3. What points would you cover?

The mother may have a second concern about leaving her son in the operating theatre. This gives you a lead to explain the preparation for theatre.

4. What points will you cover?

Finally, before leaving, reassure her that she is welcome to come to the theatre and check that she understands what will happen. Check that there are no other concerns.

(Answers on page 114)

Communication 3

A 32-year-old woman with a haemoglobin of 9 g/dl who has menorrhagia is listed for a hysterectomy. Her notes indicate she is a Jehovah's Witness.

Questions

1. What are the issues? There are at least three issues to consider.

2. How will you deal with each issue?

Communication 4 *(Answers on page 115)*

The patient is a Greek or a West Indian who is due to have an inguinal hernia repaired.

Introduce yourself and then ask about any general health problems. The patient says that he has no knowledge of any blood diseases in his family, he is well but has lost a little weight. He is a policeman. Explain the need for a sickle test. He is not keen on needles.

Questions

1. What is (are) the relevant issue(s) that may need to be discussed?

   Write down what you might expect to talk about.

2. What will you pursue now?

   He still does not want a blood test.

3. Why would he not want a blood test?

   The patient gives a history of weight loss.

4. What will you ask about?

   The patient is Sickledex-posititve.

5. How will you proceed?

Communication 5 (Answers on page 116)

You are told that the patient is having a hysterectomy and is concerned about pain relief.

Questions

1. What are the issues?
   Introduce yourself and immediately allow the patient to tell you about their problem. *"What is your anxiety?"* *"Is there a particular reason for being anxious?"*

2. *"What would you like to know about pain relief?"* What strategy will you follow for postoperative pain relief?

3. What will you explain about PCA?

4. Do intramuscular injections have a place?

5. What else will you give with the PCA?

6. What else might be given?

   Finally, you may have to help the patient choose what to have. *"What do you advise, doctor?"*

7. Your choice is . . .

Communication 6 *(Answers on page 118)*

The patient is concerned about a proposed operation for varicose veins.

Introduction – always introduce yourself by name.

This is a specific station about communication; therefore ask the patient what their concern is. Take your lead from the introductory note "is concerned".

Questions

1. What might the patient be concerned about?

In this case the patient had a tonsillectomy as a child and remembers being awake while things were being done inside the mouth.

It is not unusual for patients to mention awareness years later when they come for a second operation.

They may not have mentioned it at the time.

2. What will your response include?

3. What conditions will you try to exclude as possible reasons for what has happened?

The patient wants reassurance about this anaesthetic. They say that their mother was told that there was a fault in the apparatus last time.

4. What will you say?

Before finishing always check if there are any other concerns. In an examination it is possible to ask the actor to add another concern.

This patient says they are still frightened of dying during the anaesthetic.

5. What will you say?

Communication 7 *(Answers on page 120)*

You are asked to see a pregnant woman seeking advice about pain relief. Start with an introduction and ask what advice is required. The woman says she is anxious about having pain in labour.

Questions
1. What do you want to know?

   Patient says that she is concerned about having a lot of pain.
   She would like an epidural.

2. How will you respond?

   She wishes to know more about an epidural for labour.

3. What will you say?

   The patient decides that she wants to know about the other methods.

4. Which methods will you mention?

   The patient may be undecided and ask which technique you recommend.

5. What will you say?

Communication 8

A 10-year-old boy for an emergency appendectomy has failed to breathe at the end of the operation due to suxamethonium apnoea. You need to explain the situation to the mother.

Suggested response

The mother is distressed and anxious. Remember, people usually fear the worse.

How will you relieve anxiety? Stay calm yourself. Do not be heavy handed, take your time to establish the mother's fears and to deal with them logically and accurately. Sit the mother down and explain what has happened. Tell the truth, do not minimise the situation. Respond to her anxiety. LISTEN to what the mother is worried about and give an appropriate response.

Once the mother is calm, explain what has happened, and then what happens next. The parent will want to see the child. Do not be paternalistic. Doctors are criticised for "*I know best*" attitude. Do what the mother wants if it is reasonable, even if it is not what is done in your hospital, perhaps it should be.

Relatives usually want reassurance that their loved one is not in pain, not aware and if they will recover will they recover intact. "*Will they be alright?*"

Communication 9

You are conducting a randomised trial on a new postoperative analgesia, comparing it with morphine. You need to obtain informed consent from the patient.

What is informed consent?

Suggested response

Tell the patient the nature of the trial, what is it for and what outcomes are expected. Is a placebo involved or another drug? Explain what you are asking the patient to do, over and above their normal treatment. They need to know everything about the drug and any extra measurements or tests.

Respond to questions like, *"Can they withdraw? Does it make a difference to their treatment? What alternatives will be used if the trial drug fails? Are there any side-effects? What will be done about these side-effects if they happen?"*

Give sheet of instruction and the consent form. Allow time to read. Come back for questions and to sign consent form. Do not expect patient to sign the form without reading the instruction. Details of any payments should be explained and some trial protocols may want insurance arrangements discussed. Emphasise that treatment will be the same and they can withdraw at any time.

Confirm you will write in notes and inform surgeon and GP that they have had a trial drug and how they can contact someone afterwards if they have a worry.

Communication 10

You are with a new ODA/anaesthetic assistant. You want them to assist you with a procedure like cricoid pressure or a difficult intubation.

Suggested response

Explain cricoid pressure. Do not assume anything.

Give the purpose of the pressure. The position of the cricoid, mark it if necessary, how to press, when to press – as the patient goes to sleep as it is painful when awake, use two hands. Only release when intubated and cuff inflated, unless asked to do so before if intubation is difficult.

Difficult intubation: Have you got all the apparatus ready and working? Bougie, laryngeal mask, various tubes small and uncuffed, Magill forceps, various laryngoscope blades – Macintosh curved, long blade, straight, polio, McCoy. Keep light on from the start to make sure it does not go out.

Cricothyroid puncture if cyanosed. Or back to mask and oxygen, may need airways oral and nasal or help using mask. Call for help. (As there is no face to face contact. Explanations must be clear and accurate.)

Suction working, possibly on side if vomiting likely.

Keep cricoid pressure in place if able to ventilate.

May need drugs, atropine, glycopyrronium, and metoclopramide. Possible nasogastric tube.

Know where to find the fibreoptic laryngoscope or have it prepared ready for use.

Communication 11

You are on call and have been asked to treat a 2 year old child who is fitting in A & E.

Suggested response

You must refer to the consultant on call.
When talking to the consultant for advice or to the parents introduce yourself and explain what you want to do at each stage.
There are three aspects to the situation.

1. The assessment and resuscitation of the child.

2. The possible causes of the fitting.

3. Recognise that the parent is anxious and explain what you are doing.

1. Assessment
   Airway
   Breathing
   CVS
   IV access, if breathing lateral position and oxygen.
   Control the fitting. Diazepam IV, GA with muscle relaxants.
Assess the need for intubation to:
   Maintain oxygenation.
   Protect the airway from aspiration.
Assess the need for ventilation GCS < 9, to control hypoxia and hypercarbia, GA to control fitting or for a CT scan.
Make a rapid assessment of weight and general condition including signs of child abuse.

2. Causes
   Ask about a history of trauma, infection with sudden rise in temperature, fits in the past, drug therapy.

3. Recognise the parent's anxiety.
   Explain what is happening.
   Need for resuscitation and control of fitting.
   Ask parent for possible causes but reassure parent, who may be feeling guilty that they are responsible.
   Be guarded in the prognosis. It may be a good outcome if it is due to sudden infantile pyrexia. It may be a poor outcome if the pyrexia is due to a serious infection or a head injury. Explain that childhood fits rarely progress to adult epilepsy but epilepsy is common in the population affecting 1 in 200 people. Is there a family history of epilepsy, which may increase their anxiety? There is no evidence that epilepsy in inherited.

Communication 12

Communicating with other departments can be a challenge. The radiographer for an X-ray or the laboratory technician for a blood test. Another hospital for notes or to transfer a patient.

You are half way through a hysterectomy and a clamp has slipped and there is massive haemorrhage. Explain to the laboratory technician your need for blood when no blood has been sent for group and save.

Suggested response

Explain who you are and check you have the right department and the appropriate person. Apologise for bothering them. This is a request not a demand.

Empathy is important. Try to understand how they feel. You want a favour and they may be busy and worried about doing another test. Remember they are getting calls all the time from people who think that their problem is the most important.

Is there a protocol for massive blood loss and transfusion in the hospital that should be followed?

One procedure will be to give at least 1 litre of crystalloid and then 1 litre of colloid.

You are now asking the technician for group specific blood. Check that the technician has a group and save specimen and if not send one immediately. Do you have a blood group from the notes or a previous admission? They will want a sample of blood to confirm the group and confirm the cross match. But you are not asking for cross match blood at this moment. You will take responsibility, if necessary, for giving uncross matched blood.

Be clear what you are asking for. What is actually necessary? What are the alternatives?

You might ask for 6 or 8 units of group specific blood and two to four units of fresh frozen plasma. The plasma is to replace the protein that is not present in SAGM blood and to replace the clotting factors.

Two units of O negative blood are usually reserved for pregnant women and difficult cross-match situations.

Be realistic that there is not enough time for a full cross match. Negotiate for what you need now and call back for more, depending on the blood available in the laboratory. Remember the importance of properly labelled forms. The technician cannot help you if they have not got the correct documents. They do not want to make a mistake.

"Please" and "Thank You" are essential words in any request for a service.

Communication 13

A man is to have a colectomy but he is concerned about taking morphine, as he has been a drug addict.

Suggested response

Introduce yourself.
Identify the likely problems

1. The patient is anxious.

2. The patient has a history of drug dependency.

3. The patient needs pain relief.

1. Anxiety
   Ask the patient what they are anxious about. Do not assume that you know.
   Sympathy is showing concern. This can be demonstrated by responding with appropriate expletives like, "Oh dear. . .", "I am sorry. . .". Do not say you know how they feel. This annoys people unless you have the same problem, which you clearly do not.
   Empathy is trying to understand how the person feels. Respond by saying, "You seem to be very anxious about. . .." "That makes you feel. . ."
   Relieve anxiety by listening. Identify each problem that is causing the anxiety (there may be more than one problem). Then offer reassurance that you will deal with their problems offering help and advice.

2. Drug history
   Which drugs have or are being taken. Is the habit ongoing? The patient may try to hide the fact that they are still taking these drugs. Are there associated medical problems? Hepatitis, HIV, smoking, alcohol and related conditions?
   Do not try to wean a drug addict off their drugs. Reassure them that you will not do this.
   Determine the daily drug, dose and method of intake. Reassure the patient that they will go on receiving this regime throughout their hospital stay.

3. Pain relief
   Explore their anxieties.
   Explain all the methods of pain relief.
   Regional and all the possible local nerve blocks of relevance.
   NSAIDs and opioids with their doses and side effects.
   Explain that there is no evidence that the drug dependent patient needs a different dose of analgesia providing they continue to receive their maintenance therapy. Anxiety will increase the appreciation of pain and this needs to be reduced by explanation or short term sedatives (they may have a problem with benzodiazepines long term).

Communication 14

Case 14
You accidentally knocked a tooth out of a man when you intubated him yesterday.

Suggested response
Introduce yourself.
The likely problems are

1. The man has strong emotions and is angry.

2. There has been a complaint due to this accident.

3. What will be done to correct the problem?

1. The Anger
• Visit the patient. Do not send someone else. Do not ignore the problem.
• Sympathy. Say you are sorry. Do not apportion blame to anyone. Especially not the patient. It is not the patient's fault. Do not seek to minimise the problem.
• Empathy – try to understand how the patient is feeling. He is cross that his lovely teeth and facial expression, when he smiles, has been ruined. He may have paid a lot of money to have these teeth. He may be in pain or has bleeding gums.
• Do not look for excuses. There may have been an accident like a difficult intubation. Ask about the situation pre-operatively. Did you see the patient preoperatively? Did you discuss any loose teeth and did you write in the notes? If you did not recognise loose teeth before then why did the teeth get knocked out? Be careful how you approach this as you may come over as incompetent. If you say the intubation was difficult why did you not warn of this preoperatively or use a bougie or a laryngeal mask etc.?
• It is more honest to admit a mistake and say you are sorry and you will now do everything to make amends.
• Do not blame the patient for being a difficult patient by words or implication.

2. The complaints procedure
Go through the exact problem with the patient. If necessary have a witness. Does the patient want a witness?
Record the problem(s) in the notes and on the relevant forms and the remedy offered. You and the witness to the discussion should sign and date this record.

3. What is to be done?
Reassure that everything necessary will be done.
Either they can see their own dentist or you will personally go to see the hospital dentist and arrange an immediate referral and appointment. No

delay by waiting in a long queue.
The hospital will pay for the repair.

Finally repeat that you are very sorry that this has happened.
Discuss the problem with a consultant and the hospital complaints
department. Have a witness to all you have said. Offer to come back again to
check up.

Communication 15

You placed an epidural for labour yesterday. The mother is now complaining of headache and numbness of the upper thigh.

Suggested response
Introduce yourself.

1. See the patient. Introduce yourself and your role. Establish what is the complaint.

2. Explain the possible causes.

3. If this is post-lumbar puncture headache explain how this will be managed.

1. Establish the complaint.
Be sympathetic.
Do not assume this headache is post-lumbar puncture without discussing all the details. Where is the headache? Is it occipital and frontal? Is it affected by position?
Is there neck stiffness, a problem with vision or any other neurological problem?

2. Consider all causes of headache, post-lumbar puncture headache, pre-eclampsia, intracranial haemorrhage, infection, tension headache and migraine.
Where is the numbness in the leg. Is there leg weakness?
Were there any of these problems present before the epidural?

The numbness of the thigh. Is it nerve root or peripheral nerve distribution?
Is it related to the epidural or to an abdominal wall nerve praxia.

3. Relevant treatment for post-lumbar puncture headache.
Explain that it is not life threatening but a great inconvenience. It is limited to 7 to 14 days.
Two way forwards. Explain both.
* Bed rest, lying flat most of the time. Analgesia and laxatives.
* Blood patch. Repeat the epidural and then inject 20-30 ml of the patient's own blood to seal the hole by pressure of clot or a fibrin web. They can then usually walk with no headache within 1 hour. No effect on future epidurals.

Communication 16

Giving advice to another doctor.

You have been approached, by a medical registrar, about admitting a patient to HDU.

The patient has a history of being admitted 3 days ago with breathlessness. The patient has deteriorated and the pulse oximeter reading is 89% breathing 60% oxygen. The BP is 75/55, heart rate is 140/minute.

What advice will you give?

Suggested response

Introduce yourself.
You must see the patient and record your findings and the advice given.
Ask the doctor what the results of his/her history and examination have been? You may get some information from the other doctor but it is essential to see the sick patient yourself.
What aspects of the patient are you particularly interested in?

1. You want to know about the initial assessment of
* Airway, breathing, pulse, and conscious level. If the patient is exhausted they will be sleeping or not rousable.
* Does the patient need intubation to protect the airway from hypoxia or aspiration?
* Does the patient need ventilation to control their oxygenation and carbon dioxide?
* Have they become exhausted and developed respiratory failure with inability to clear their secretions?

2. You will discuss a differential diagnosis
Explain the likely causes
* Respiratory causes – sepsis, aspiration, and bronchospasm with dehydration, pneumothorax, and cancer.
* Cardiovascular causes – heart failure with or without fluid depletion or overload. Fluid loss – haemorrhage, vomiting or diarrhoea.
* Endocrine diseases – diabetes, myxoedema and Addisonian crisis.
* Metabolic acidosis.
* Drug overdose.
* Others. Septicaemia, carcinomatosis.

Does the patient need ITU admission?
Indications are the need for
* Tracheal intubation. To control the airway, clear secretions.
* Mechanical Ventilation. To control the blood gases.
* Oxygenation may be achieved by
  * An increase inspired oxygen tension with CPAP.

- More than routine IV access and simple monitoring. CVP, arterial line for blood gases, cardiac output assessment.

Check
- Bladder catheter for urine output. With a low BP it is unlikely that urine will be produced but successful resuscitation will be reflected in the urine volume.
- IV Fluids and a vasoconstrictor may be required.
- A pulmonary flotation catheter and pulmonary capillary wedge pressure may be required to assess cardiac output, pulmonary pressures and vascular resistance and guide therapy.
- If IPPV is contemplated it is important that there is the means to raise the BP as the increased intrathoracic pressure will reduce cardiac filling, particularly if the CVP is low in a dehydrated patient.

Answers
Communication

Answers – Communication 1

Relative's scenario: Play the part of a person whose spouse has been admitted following a cerebral haemorrhage and whose life is only supported by a ventilator.

You want to know if s/he is dead.

1. What does the person already know? What do they want explained?

2. *a.* Brain death tests and turning off the ventilator. The involvement of the relative in the decision to turn off a ventilator is difficult. The turning off of a ventilator is a medical decision. The relative does not have medical knowledge, but they do have feelings, which in these circumstances are confused. In grief the relative will not necessarily be able to make rational decisions. For one partner to die is a threat to the very existence of the remaining partner who is not going to want to be put into the situation of turning off their own life. The reasons for turning off have to be explained to the relative.
   b. Potential donor – card carrier.
   c. Refer the case to the coroner.

3. Explain the procedures for brain death tests, in the presence of a known diagnosis. Stop all drugs. Normal body chemistry and temperature. A series of tests of brain function. All tests done by two doctors. No pupil movement, no eye movement, no spontaneous breathing, no response to pain. If no response present then all tests repeated. Explain peripheral movements due to spinal reflexes.

4. Deal with the possibility of the patient being a donor. Is s/he a potential donor?

   Was s/he in good health? The question of testing for HIV and hepatitis should be mentioned. Did s/he carry a donor card or express any wish? Indicate the organs that might be used: kidney, heart, lungs, liver, pancreas, corneas. Perhaps introduce the idea that someone else may be helped out of their tragedy.

5. Explain the role of the coroner in establishing cause of death, when death is sudden or suspicious. Some coroners will want to be informed when donation is involved or if there has been an industrial disease. Explain that the coroner may want to talk to them. Reassure them that this is not a court of law, s/he is not looking for blame.

Answers – Communication 2

Parent scenario   You are a parent of a child who is to have an operation. You are worried about his anaesthetic as your nephew had a tonsillectomy and needed ventilation for some 3 hours postoperatively. You know that it was something to do with a muscle relaxant called suxamethonium. A second issue is that you want to know what will happen on the day of surgery.

1. Previous operations with complications; congenital or acquired conditions; family illness or death; present condition.

2. Inherited conditions that might present in childhood (not many children have acquired diseases in early life). Suxamethonium apnoea, porphyria, malignant hyperpyrexia and congenital conditions of CVS, CNS and cystic fibrosis. Trauma associated with an accident. Anaphylactic conditions are rare in children. A relative overdose of local anaesthetic or opiate are possibilities. Establish exactly what happened. If it was a congenital condition is there a blood relationship to this child?

3. Explain the nature of suxamethonium, commonly used to secure the airway.

   Defective gene inherited from mother and father which then leads to a failure to produce the normal enzyme needed to destroy this drug quickly. There is a slower route for elimination of the drug, hence the 3-hour delay in recovery.

   Treatment: maintain respiratory support and sleep while recovery occurs. If there is concern about this child, he and other members of the family need testing for the presence of pseudocholinesterase. Give the incidence of the atypical gene (3:10,000) and explain that it runs in families but may not affect her child. If necessary you will not give suxamethonium or mivacurium.

   Other possible scenarios but associated with a longer recovery and residual effects would be: The relative might have presented with abdominal pain, had an appendicectomy which was normal, but the abdominal pain was a presentation of porphyria or diabetes. If porphyria: establish a blood relationship and whether other family members are affected. Porphyria can be difficult to diagnose unless the person is having an attack. There are a limited number of drugs that are relatively safe to give. These include: muscle relaxants, opioids, nitrous oxide, volatile agents, local anaesthetics and benzodiazepines.

   Malignant hyperpyrexia (MH) is rare, even in children (1:14,000). Any relative of a MH patient should be investigated at a specialist centre by exposing a muscle biopsy to caffeine or halothane.

   Anaphylaxis. If a person is likely to be allergic to a drug, skin tests are used to try to define which drugs should be avoided.

4. You will see her child: general health and development, look for loose teeth, assess airway and a possible venous access. EMLA cream, possible oral premedication.

Fluids to drink up to 2 hours before the operation. Come to theatre in any clothes, with toy, with one parent to the anaesthetic room. Attach monitors, either a venous or inhalation induction, whichever seems appropriate depending on the ease of venous access and airway. Once the child is asleep, the parent will leave with a nurse.

Explain postoperative pain relief, opioids, NSAI, suppositories and local anaesthesia if relevant and return to drinking. Indicate that the mother can come to the recovery room.

Answers – Communication 3

Patient's scenario   Play the part of a Jehovah's Witness requiring a hysterectomy for menorhagia.

1. A Jehovah's Witness is likely to have a particular belief about blood transfusion. Determine what these beliefs are. In particular, what is their attitude to donated blood and donated blood products like FFP, albumin, pre-donated blood, autologous blood transfusion and cell salvage, the use of autologous blood and cardiac surgery with a bypass pump?

   Be explicit in clarifying the issues: *"Am I correct in assuming you would rather die than receive…?"* *"Would you be happy with…?"*

   Get all the details written down. What is acceptable and what is not to be given. Use a suitable consent form.

   If the case is difficult there are a number of doctors and hospitals willing to treat such patients and transfer can be arranged.

   Pre-treatment.

   Is the operation life-saving – how urgent is it? Is there a place for iron and folic acid therapy or erythropoetin preoperatively?

2. Limiting blood loss. Various techniques are available for limiting blood loss. Discuss hypotensive anaesthetic techniques, the use of local vasoconstrictor and above all strict haemostasis. It is the surgeon who usually causes blood loss not the anaesthetist. Monitoring might well involve direct BP measurement. Explain the modified Allen's test.

   Be aware of the ASA guidelines on blood replacement. Above 10 g/dl blood is almost never needed, below 6 g/dl it is often needed.

   If the Hb falls very low – below 4 or 3 gm/dl – then at the end of the operation it would be wise to continue to ventilate in an ITU. This will limit oxygen demand by good pain relief, stopping shivering and reducing muscle activity. It will also prevent pulmonary oedema if the plasma protein concentration is low. Ventilation for a few days will allow the Hb and plasma proteins to regenerate and bring the oxygen delivery back to normal limits.

Answers – Communication 4

Patient's scenario Play the part of a Greek, Indian or African who might have sickle or thalassaemia but has also lost some weight. You work as a policeman. You are frightened of doctors and needles.

1. Mediterranean patients and those from Africa, or of African descent, have the possibility of having sickle cell disease or thalassaemia. Approximately 25% of Africans carry the sickle cell gene. Sickle cell disease is also prevalent in certain parts of India and the Far East.

2. Four issues:
   a. The weight loss, in the absence of symptoms. Has he got a chronic infection – hepatitis, tuberculosis; a cancer; metabolic disorder such as diabetes?
   b. Why is he frightened of needles? You might offer a small needle and EMLA cream.
   c. The inguinal hernia can be associated with an intra-abdominal tumour.
   d. Always ask about occupation. How might it be relevant?

3. He may fear a test revealing a disease which would exclude him from his job such as hepatitis, epilepsy, AIDS, illegal drugs – steroids for sports or recreational drugs, high alcohol intake.

   How will you deal with this?

   Indicate that the test is only for sickle cell disease. Is he frightened of being tested for anything else? It might be important to know if he has other diseases such as AIDS or hepatitis. Reassure him that nothing else is tested without his consent, if it is not relevant to the present condition.

4. How much weight has he lost and over how many weeks? Is it deliberate: is he on a diet? Ask about any other symptoms such as malaise, tiredness, pyrexia or lumps. Think of infection, cancer or diabetes.

5. The sickledex test does not differentiate trait from disease. The blood should be tested by electrophoreses and if the disease is present consider a local anaesthetic technique – epidural or spinal. Avoid tourniquets. Check whether there is a contraindication such as a clotting problem, back infection and obtain consent. Then be prepared to explain the details of an epidural: IV access and fluids with BP monitoring, position, risk 1:100 of post-spinal tap headache. Leg weakness and numbness, retention of urine.

Answers – Communication 5

Patient's scenario Play the part of a patient who is to have abdominal surgery and is anxious to have good pain relief.

1. This is a scenario about postoperative pain relief. The patient may have experienced pain in previous operations. Do not wander off into other areas without dealing with this worry first.

2. This requires a logical method of explanation. *"There are many different methods of relieving pain, do you want to know about all of them?"* Balanced analgesia should include: opioids as PCA or IM, local anaesthetics, NSAIDs, entonox, transcutaneous nerve stimulation (TENS).

3. What will you say about PCA?

   Explain how it works. You press a button and the device gives you a small dose. You can titrate the total dose against your pain and any side-effects. Side-effects: some sedation, nausea and vomiting – you will have an anti-emetic. Because the peaks in the doses are less, the nausea and itch (if it occurs) should be less severe.

   There is a short lock out of up to 10 minutes before taking another dose, to give the previous dose time to work. So you cannot give yourself too much, nor can you become addicted. Only you should press the button.

4. Intramuscular injections are still used. *"There may be nausea which can usually be treated with an anti-emetic. If you require a limited number of doses this is a method to consider. If you prefer the nurse to give you pain relief, then you can call the nurse or they will come and ask you if you have any pain and give you an appropriate dose of morphine when you ask. Do not keep quiet and suffer in silence, make sure you ask the nurse for a dose when you need it, you will not become addicted."*

   Intramuscular drugs are best given by the nurse asking the patient every hour whether or not they have pain. Reassure the patient that nausea will be dealt with and addiction is not a problem.

5. Give an anti-inflammatory drug. This can be given as a wafer onto the tongue, as a suppository, or by injection. There are a number of conditions when non-steroidal anti-inflammatory drugs may not be advisable and there is a need to check that the patient does not have: peptic ulcers, renal impairment, asthma with nasal polyps, liver disease, or a clotting problem. *"I will give you a dose of non-steroidal before you wake up. These drugs are good as the sole analgesic after any severe pain is easing and when you can take oral medication."*

   Obtain informed consent before using a suppository and warn about anal discharge. Record your advice in the patient's notes.

6. Local anaesthetics, particularly if the patient has a problem with opioids or NSAIDs.

   There are a number of different local anaesthetic techniques that can be used, either single dose, top ups or continuous infusions to give longer relief.

   Explain that: *"Normally a dose of local anaesthetic is placed into and around the wound before you wake up. This will make it numb for a few hours. Consider an epidural. There are more potential problems than with the other techniques and it requires more intensive nursing postoperatively."*

   "An epidural can be continued into the postoperative period but the legs may be numb and weak and the bladder may not function normally. There is a risk of a headache due to a dural tap and low CSF pressure. The blood pressure can go down so you need a drip; we have to be careful to observe your breathing closely after the operation and you may get an itch if an opioid is mixed with the local anaesthetic."

   If you are thinking of an epidural do not forget to warn the patient of headache incidence (1 : 100), bladder weakness and retention of urine and, if using opioids, respiratory problems and itch.

7. Find out which one the patient might prefer.

   If they do not know, offer your best method. *"I would recommend a balanced method: an anti-inflammatory and opioid drug while you are asleep and local anaesthetic into the wound before you wake up. A PCA device with an anti-emetic once you are awake enough to press the button."*

   The test is to cover all the information in an organised way.

Answers – Communication 6

Patient's scenario Play the part of patient who was aware during a childhood tonsillectomy and is to have a varicose vein operation. You are also frightened of dying during a general anaesthetic.

1. Concern might be about awareness, fear of not waking up or death, nausea and vomiting, pain. Whatever the concern is, ask why? Has something affected them, a relative or friend?

2. *a.* Show some sympathy.
   b. Find out when the awareness happened. Patients may remember the intubation if there is a delay and the effect of induction agents is passing off.

   Think – was this a difficult intubation?
   c. The patient may be aware during the operation for various reasons. Emergency situations such as severe hypotension may mean 100% oxygen was given. There may have been a faulty anaesthetic machine, ventilator or a vaporiser became empty. The later implies a lack of monitoring.
   d. It may have happened in recovery if there was a problem with the airway postoperatively. Ascertain whether the patient could move or were they paralysed?
   e. Were they in pain or did they hear a conversation?

   Impress on everyone that you are taking the situation seriously, getting all the facts. Have they had any subsequent operations with or without problems?

3. Try to exclude an anaphylaxis reaction – do you have an 'alert' disc for an allergy? If the awareness was in recovery was the anaesthetic prolonged and why? Exclude a suxamethonium apnoea ventilated without sedation. Indicate that you will send for the notes of his operation.

4. How will you proceed with this operation?
   a. Would you consider a local anaesthetic for this operation? Before committing yourself to a local anaesthetic make sure that there are no contraindications: patient willing, anatomy not abnormal, no coagulation problems, no sepsis.
   b. An amnesic premedication before this operation.
   c. If a general anaesthetic: Reassure that you will stay with patient all the time.
   Full monitoring including anaesthetic agent concentration. Avoid paralysis or use minimum paralysis so that patient can indicate awareness.

5. Determine the cause for concern. Is there a reason for the fear? Their mother died during an anaesthetic. If possible find the medical notes.

What were the circumstances? Is there a link? You are seeking a precise explanation.

It may be necessary to exclude an inherited or an allergic condition. Has anyone else in the patient's family died or been abnormally ill following an anaesthetic?

Have you excluded suxamethonium apnoea, anaphylaxis, or rare conditions such as: porphyria, malignant hyperpyrexia, or cardiomyopathy?

In other cases when awareness is reported check that it is true awareness.

Answers – Communication 7

Patient's scenario   Play the part of a pregnant woman who is concerned about pain relief in labour. You want an epidural but have had attacks of abdominal pain, suggesting an abruption.

1. Why is she anxious? Has she had a previous painful labour, or has a relative or friend had pain? What does she know about pain relief and has she got an opinion as to what she wants?

2. Do not fall into the trap of offering an epidural without checking the obstetric history.

   Ask about:
   - Number of weeks pregnant.
   - History of bleeding.
   - Previous caesarean section.
   - Back operations.
   - Pain or deformity.
   - Neurological condition especially multiple sclerosis.
   - Back infection.
   - Blood coagulation problem.

3. Explain what an epidural involves: an intravenous infusion in case of fall in blood pressure, lie on side or sit up, injection and catheter to back. Problems with hypotension, loss of bladder control, leg weakness, and loss of sensation below waist. Often a shortened first stage but prolonged second stage. Headache if dural puncture 1:100. It may not be possible if the anatomy is difficult, bleeding indicates abruption or placenta praevia, or pain indicating abruption.

4. You should be prepared to discuss a range of analgesic techniques including: TENS, relaxation, entonox, intramuscular and intravenous analgesia and PCA when epidural analgesia is not possible.

   Obstetric analgesia is about pain relief in labour not just an epidural service.

5. You may have to give advantages and disadvantages or an opinion.

   Think of issues such as: would an epidural be an advantage to the mother or baby – does she have diabetes, heart condition, pre eclampsia, or is there a multiple pregnancy, breech or premature baby?

   What are the person's expectations about severity of pain. Local anaesthetics are the only technique to completely remove pain but some mothers feel disappointed that they have not had real labour, others may not want the side-effects. The options can be left open.

RESUSCITATION

4

There will almost certainly be a resuscitation station in the Anaesthetic OSCE Examination. This can be basic or advanced life support for a child or adult, under circumstance such as myocardial collapse, trauma, choking, drowning and electrocution or during pregnancy. In order to pass a resuscitation examination it is necessary to learn the current protocols by heart and follow them exactly. If you do not learn them and do not apply them exactly, marks are lost unnecessarily.

The protocols produced here are those that can be found on the UK Resuscitation Council web site www.resus.org.uk. They are also published, with some variations, in the journal *Resuscitation* 2000; 46: 1–448.

The reasons for rigid protocols are:

a. The management of cardiac arrests is a team effort, often carried out by people with different training backgrounds and in difficult circumstances. It is most efficient if all members of the team are following the same system.
b. Cardiac arrests are very stressful, especially for less experienced members of the team. A protocol helps everyone to keep their mind on what comes next.

There is not a lot of thought required to carry out a protocol. You do need to remember the SAFETY of yourself and the team. For basic life support, a scenario may involve personal danger. A patient may have been electrocuted. Do not put your own life at risk. Remove the source of danger first. Remember to be safe in using a defibrillator, which can put others at risk.

Basic Life Support

Points to remember
1. Follow the **guidelines exactly,** do not take short cuts and miss points out.
2. Remember safety. Only approach the patient when you have checked it is safe to do so. Do not rush in.
3. When to go for help. As a rule, **go for help before starting resuscitation**. If the patient is not breathing, go for help immediately. Do not start resuscitation or feel for a heart beat unless it is a child. The **exception** is if there is a primary respiratory arrest due to trauma or drowning then give 1 minute of basic life support. Then go for help.

4. Practice on a manikin as much as possible.
5. Wear sensible clothes.

Lay people are now encouraged to look for signs of life for 10 seconds, and not waste time trying to feel for a pulse they may never find. Professionals should know where to feel for a carotid pulse.

The ratio of chest compression to ventilation should be 15:2 whether one or more people are working on the patient. If the patient is intubated, chest compression should continue at the same time as ventilation. A laryngeal mask airway or Combitube are alternatives to a tracheal tube.

Advanced life support
Apply the protocols with an emphasis on safety, particularly when using the defibrillator. There is time, do not rush.

The main changes that have been introduced recently are:

High dose epinephrine is not recommended. Give epinephrine 1 mg IV or 2–3 mg into the tracheal tube. VF consider: Amiodarone 300 mg diluted in 20 ml dextrose IV, followed by 150 mg and an infusion of 1 mg/min for 6 hours to maximum of 2 g. Magnesium 8 mmol if there is a deficiency. Lidocaine should not be given if amiodarone has been given but can be given alone 30 mg/min to 17 mg/kg. Procainamide is an alternative. Bretylium is not recommended. Bicarbonate may be given if the pH is < 7.1 (H$^+$ >80 mmol/l) or if arrest associated with a tricyclic overdose or hyperkalaemia.

Asystole
CPR and first dose of epinephrine 1 mg, atropine 3 mg IV or 6 mg in 10 ml into the tracheal tube.

Pulseless electrical activity
CPR and epinephrine 1 mg every 3 minutes, no more. Then atropine 3 mg IV or 6 mg into the tracheal tube.

Use of the defibrillator
The treatment of ventricular fibrillation detected by wide, bizarre, fast QRS complexes on the ECG requires the use of a defibrillator. An examiner will want to know that you are competent in its use.

1. Switch on ECG.
2. Connect ECG red to right shoulder, yellow to left shoulder, green anywhere.
3. Switch on defibrillator.
4. Check rhythm on Lead II.
5. Pads to chest. These may be replicas but should be placed in the correct place. Right sternum and apex. Avoid ECG electrodes and other items on the chest such as GTN patches. Place the paddles firmly on the patient's chest.
6. Place defibrillator paddles onto the pads.
7. Stand clear before charging. Look carefully around the bed to make sure no one, including yourself is touching it. Say, "Stand clear".

8. Oxygen away.
9. Output 200 J check. Dial the required energy level. In adults, 200 J is used first as the device charges to 200 quickly and gives little myocardial damage, a second 200 J is used, as the first shock will reduce transthoracic impedance, then 360 J. Make sure it is in synchronous mode. The interval between each shock is about 1 minute or four cycles of 15:2 resuscitation.
10. Charge. Only charge the paddles when they are on the patient. **Do not wave** the charged paddles through the air.
11. Shock.
12. Check the ECG display. Leave the paddles on the chest ready for the next shock if there is a shockable rhythm. Do not wave them about. If rhythm returns to normal ask the assistant to turn the defibrillator off. **Do not wave** the paddles through the air when the defibrillator is on.

In addition to demonstrating the basic skills you may be asked questions on the treatment of various dysrhythmias. The majority of marks will usually be awarded for the proper demonstration of basic or advanced life support skills.

You should know how to follow a protocol for resuscitating a child and a pregnant mother. A pregnant mother should be resuscitated by tilting her towards one side with a wedge, pillow or any other support to displace the uterus off the mid line. It is logical to tip towards the left to take pressure off the vena cava but, if this is not effective, tip in the other direction or gently, manually push the uterus to one side with the palm of the hand.

The choking adult should be slapped on the back. If this fails, use a Heimlick manouevre. An adult is approached from behind. The arms are brought round the abdomen and the hands clenched together under the xiphisternum. The hands are then forced in and upwards as if trying to wind the patient to increase the intrathoracic pressure below the obstruction.

A choking child is held upside down and slapped on the back.

Resuscitation 1 (*Answers on page 127*)

Questions
What are the steps in resuscitation and how are they performed?

(Answers on page 128)

Resuscitation 2

Question
How should CPR be performed?

Resuscitation 3
(Answers on page 129)

Questions

1. What is your procedure, in a logical order, for using the debrillator safely?

2. How will you resuscitate a drowned, trauma or pregnant patient?

Answers
Resuscitation

Answers – Resuscitation 1

- Look for electric wires or other electrical cause of fibrillation. Turn off at mains before approaching the patient.
- Shake the patient to ask, "Are you alright?"
- Shout for help.
- Check the
  - **Airway** – with care of the neck, finger sweep of mouth to clear
  - **Breathing** – listen and feel for 5 seconds
  - **Circulation** – feel for a carotid pulse for 5 seconds.
- Go for help.

Answer – Resuscitation 2

CPR for an adult

Chest compression should be with two hands placed over the lower third of the sternum in the mid line. Depress 4–5 cm at a rate of 60–80 per minute. The ratio of compression to ventilation should be 15:2 for one or more operators. Each breath should aim to give 800–1200 ml taking 1 second for inspiration and 2 for expiration. If the patient is intubated, do not try to synchronise ventilation with chest compression.

CPR in children

Do not use a finger sweep as more damage may be caused, care of loose teeth.

If there is no breathing, give 5 breaths then feel for the pulse. This may be easier in the brachial artery. If no pulse, if the child is under 1-year-old use a heart rate of 100 bpm, and over 1 year 60 bpm, with a ratio to breathing of 5:1.

Chest compression should use two fingers, one finger breadth below a line joining the nipples and depress 2 cm. In the older child, use the heel of the hand 2 cm above the xiphisternum and depress 3 cm. After 20 cycles call for the emergency services.

Ventilation

To ventilate an adult, compress the nose and blow a maximum breath into the lungs through the mouth. In a child under 1 year the adult mouth fits over the mouth and nose. Sufficient volume is forced into the child's mouth to see the chest rise. In a small child this may be the volume in the adult's mouth. The adult should take a normal breath each time to maintain a high oxygen content in the exhaled or dead space gas. It is easy to distend the stomach as the resistance of the trachea and the oesophagus are similar in small children. If the costal margin is lost then a catheter should be passed to empty the stomach.

Answer – Resuscitation 3

1. Defibrillator procedure

- Administer a mechanical defibrillation shock by thumping the precordium if present at the time of the collapse or no defibrillator available.
- If no pulse or ventricular fibrillation on ECG, use the defibrillator.
- ECG set at LEAD II for P wave.
- Turn defibrillator on.
- Check rhythm.
- Apply paddles.
- Stand clear.
- Oxygen away.
- Output to 200 J.
- Charge.
- Shock.
- Look at ECG for rhythm and feel pulse.
  (Intubate, establish IV access and give epinephrine 1 mg.)
- Re-commence CPR. Allow 1 minute or 4 x 15:2 between shocks.

Administer further shocks of 200 J and 360 J. An initial 200 J is used because it produces little myocardial damage. The second 200 J is used because the first shock will reduce transthoracic impedance.

Remember to keep the paddles on the chest and never wave them in the air if they are charged.

Ask assistant to turn defibrillator off before transferring paddles directly to device when finished.

2. a. Drowned or trauma patient
- Safe approach. Shout for help.
- Check response to painful stimulus.
- Open airway.
- Head tilt and chin lift.
- Jaw thrust in trauma.
- Breathing – listen for sound at mouth, feel mouth for damp, warm air on hand.
- Look at chest for movement **for not more than 10 seconds**.
- If no response, **5 ventilation breaths**.
- Check for pulse **10 seconds**.
- No response. **CPR for 1 minute**.
- **Ratio chest compression:respiration 15:2**.
- Then **Go for help**.

b. Pregnant mother
- CPR **with a wedge or manual displacement of uterus sideways**.
- Use anything to make a wedge, pillow, rolled up coat.
- Place a wedge under the right side to move the uterus off the vena

cava. If the cardiac output is still low try a wedge under the left side or gently push the uterus over with the palm of the hand. The same principle can apply to any space-occupying lesion in the abdomen pressing on the vena cava in the supine position.

Self-test 1: Adult Basic Life Support

(Answer on page 141)

Complete the algorithm.

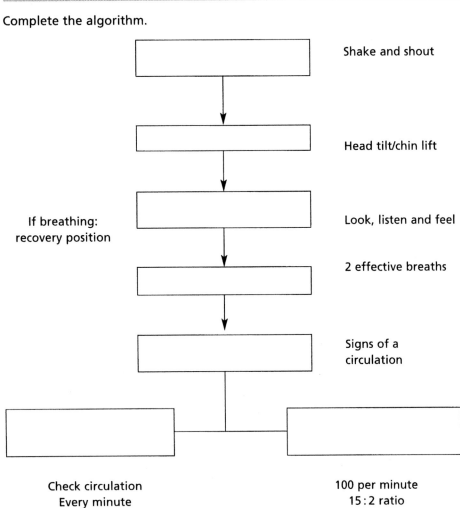

Shake and shout

Head tilt/chin lift

If breathing:
recovery position

Look, listen and feel

2 effective breaths

Signs of a
circulation

Check circulation
Every minute

100 per minute
15 : 2 ratio

Send or go for help as soon as possible according to guidelines:

Self-test 2: Adult Advanced Life Support

(Answer on page 142)

Complete the algorithm.

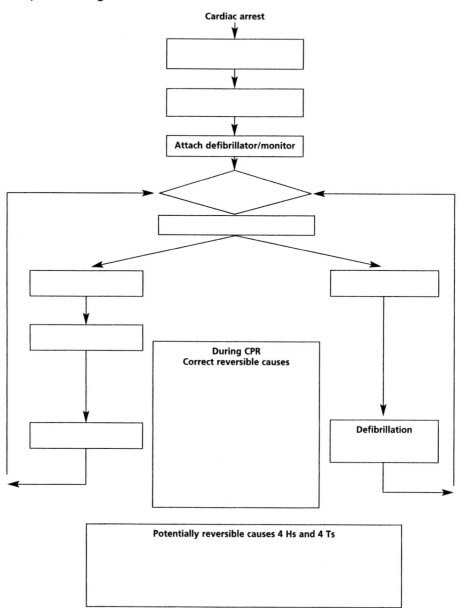

Cardiac arrest

Attach defibrillator/monitor

During CPR
Correct reversible causes

Defibrillation

Potentially reversible causes 4 Hs and 4 Ts

(*Answer on page 143*)

Self-test 3: Paediatric Basic Life Support

Complete the algorithm.

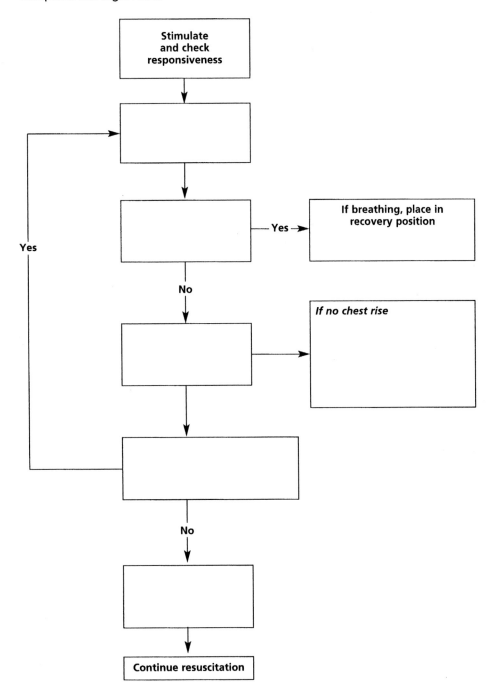

Self-test 4: Paediatric Advanced Life Support

(Answer on page 144)

Complete the algorithm.

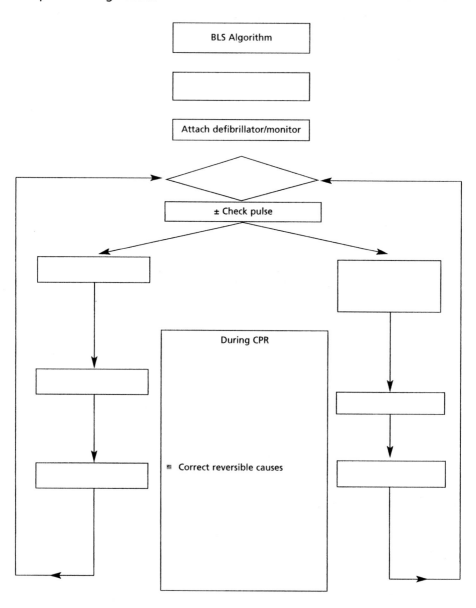

(Answer on page 145)

Self-test 5: Pulseless electrical activity

Question
Complete the protocol for an adult with pulseless electrical activity.

Consider and treat:

1. _____

2. _____

3. _____

4. _____

5. _____

6. _____

7. _____

Then:

8. _____ + _____ (if not already)

9. _____

10. _____

Self-test 6: Bradycardia *(Answer on page 146)*

Complete the algorithm.

(Includes rate inappropriately slow for haemodynamic state)
If appropriate, give oxygen and establish IV access

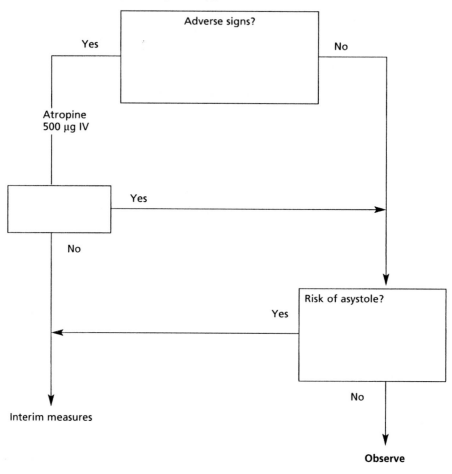

Atropine
500 µg IV

Interim measures

Observe

Seek expert help

Self-test 7: Broad Complex Tachycardia

(Answer on page 147)

Complete the algorithm.

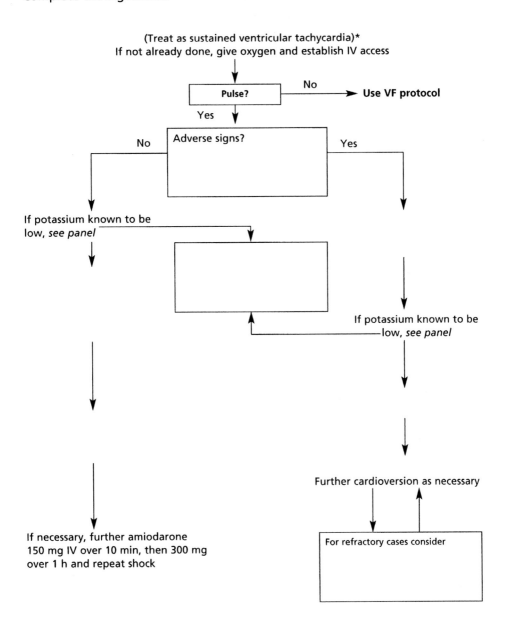

(Treat as sustained ventricular tachycardia)*
If not already done, give oxygen and establish IV access

Pulse?

No → **Use VF protocol**

Yes

Adverse signs?

No   Yes

If potassium known to be low, *see panel*

If potassium known to be low, *see panel*

Further cardioversion as necessary

If necessary, further amiodarone 150 mg IV over 10 min, then 300 mg over 1 h and repeat shock

For refractory cases consider

Doses throughout are based on an adult of average body weight.
*For paroxysms of tosades de pointes, use magnesium as above or overdrive pacing (expert help strongly recommended).
†DC shock is always given under sedation/general anaesthesia.

Self-test 8: Narrow Complex Tachycardia

(Answer on page 148)

Complete the algorithm.

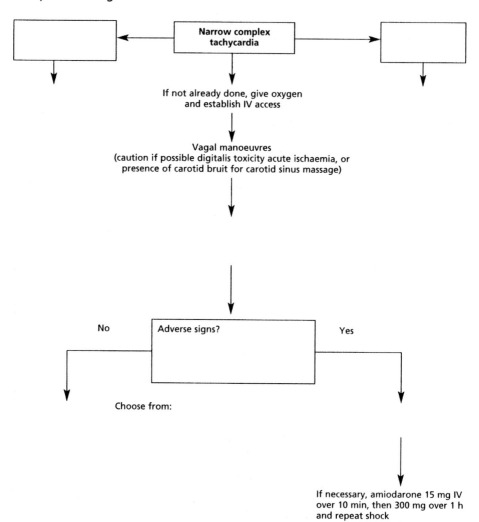

If not already done, give oxygen
and establish IV access

Vagal manoeuvres
(caution if possible digitalis toxicity acute ischaemia, or
presence of carotid bruit for carotid sinus massage)

Adverse signs?

No   Yes

Choose from:

If necessary, amiodarone 15 mg IV
over 10 min, then 300 mg over 1 h
and repeat shock

Doses throughout are based on an adult of average body weight.
A starting dose of 6 mg adenosine is currently outside the UK license for this agent.
*Theophylline and related compounds block the effect of adenosine. Patients on dipyridamole, carbamazepine, or with denervated hearts have a marked exaggerated effect which may be hazardous.
†DC shock is always given under sedation/general anaesthesia.
‡Not to be used in patients receiving beta-blockers.

(Answer on page 149)

Self-test 9: Newborn Life Support

Complete the algorithm.

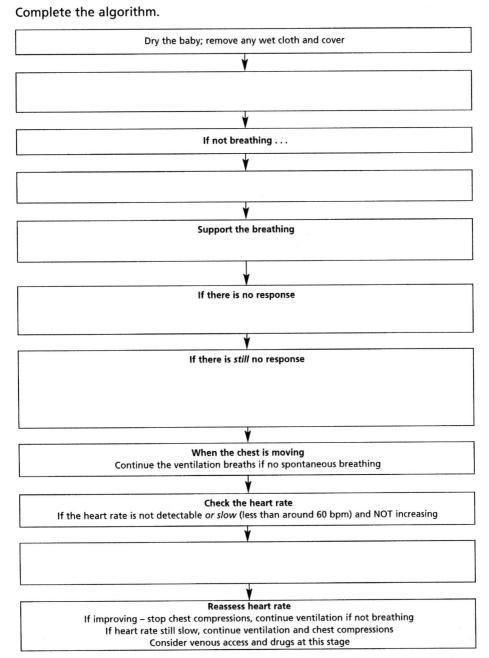

Dry the baby; remove any wet cloth and cover

If not breathing . . .

Support the breathing

If there is no response

If there is *still* no response

When the chest is moving
Continue the ventilation breaths if no spontaneous breathing

Check the heart rate
If the heart rate is not detectable *or slow* (less than around 60 bpm) and NOT increasing

Reassess heart rate
If improving – stop chest compressions, continue ventilation if not breathing
If heart rate still slow, continue ventilation and chest compressions
Consider venous access and drugs at this stage

AT ALL STAGES, ASK. DO YOU NEED HELP?
In the presence of meconium remember: Screaming babies have an open airway.
Floppy babies: have a look.

Answer – Self-test 1: Adult Basic Life Support

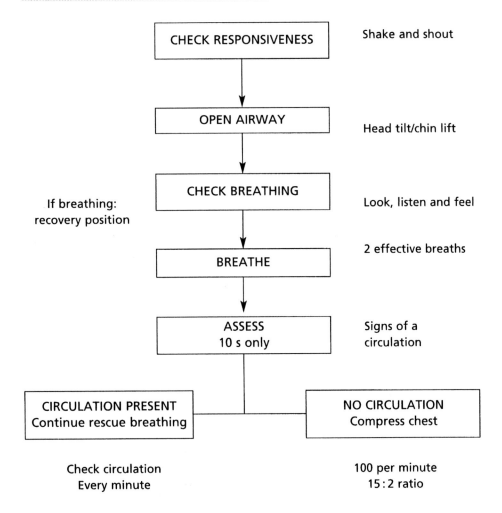

CHECK RESPONSIVENESS — Shake and shout

OPEN AIRWAY — Head tilt/chin lift

CHECK BREATHING — Look, listen and feel

If breathing: recovery position

BREATHE — 2 effective breaths

ASSESS 10 s only — Signs of a circulation

CIRCULATION PRESENT Continue rescue breathing

NO CIRCULATION Compress chest

Check circulation Every minute

100 per minute 15 : 2 ratio

Send or go for help as soon as possible according to guidelines:

Answer – Self-test 2: Adult Advanced Life Support

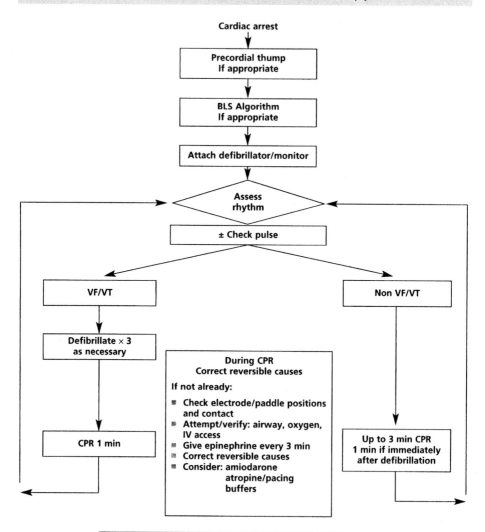

Cardiac arrest

Precordial thump
If appropriate

BLS Algorithm
If appropriate

Attach defibrillator/monitor

Assess rhythm

± Check pulse

VF/VT

Non VF/VT

Defibrillate × 3 as necessary

During CPR
Correct reversible causes

If not already:

- Check electrode/paddle positions and contact
- Attempt/verify: airway, oxygen, IV access
- Give epinephrine every 3 min
- Correct reversible causes
- Consider: amiodarone
  atropine/pacing
  buffers

CPR 1 min

Up to 3 min CPR
1 min if immediately after defibrillation

Potentially reversible causes 4 Hs and 4 Ts

Hypoxia
Hypovolaemia
Hyper/hypokalaemia and metabolic disorders
Hypothermia
Tension pneumothorax
Tamponade
Toxic/therapeutic disturbances
Thromboembolic/mechanical obstruction

Answer – Self-test 3: Paediatric Basic Life Support

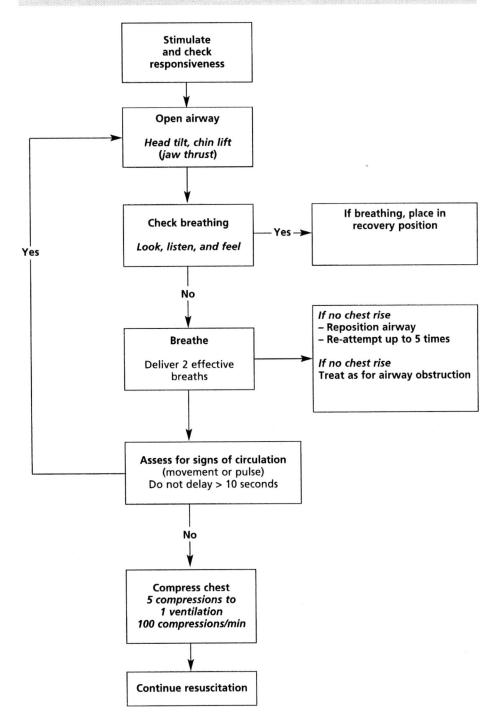

Answer – Self-test 4: Paediatric Advanced Life Support

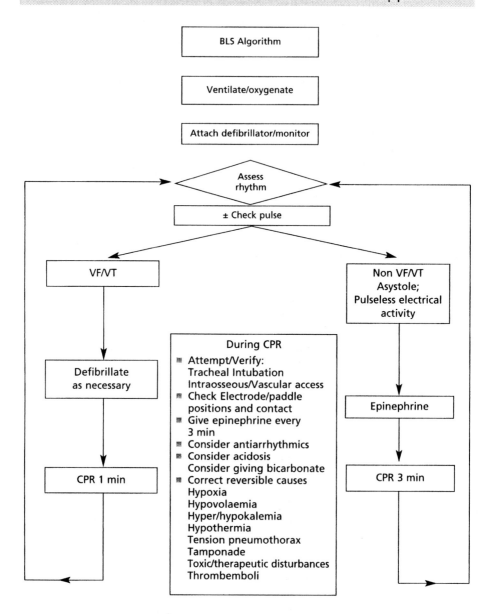

Answer – Self test 5: Pulseless electrical activity

Consider and treat:

1. Hypovolaemia

2. Hypothermia

3. Tension pneumothorax

4. Cardiac tamponade

5. Drug overdose

6. Electrolyte imbalance

7. Pulmonary embolus

Then:

8. Intubate   + IV access   (if not already) ◄─┐

9. 1 mg epinephrine   │

10. CPR sequences 15:2 × 10   ─────────────────────►─┘

Answer – Self-test 6: Bradycardia

(Includes rate inappropriately slow for haemodynamic state)
If appropriate, give oxygen and establish IV access

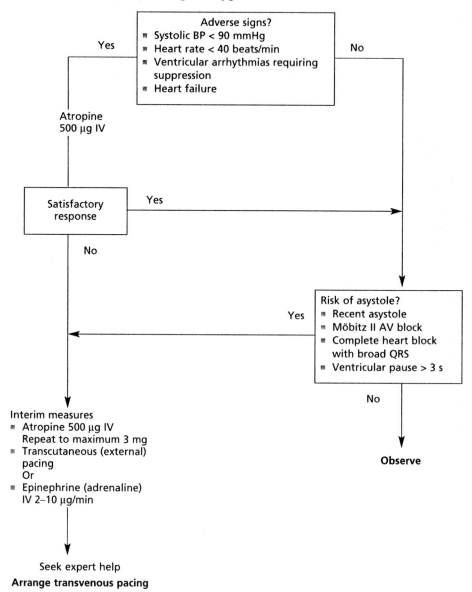

Answer – Self-test 7: Broad Complex Tachycardia

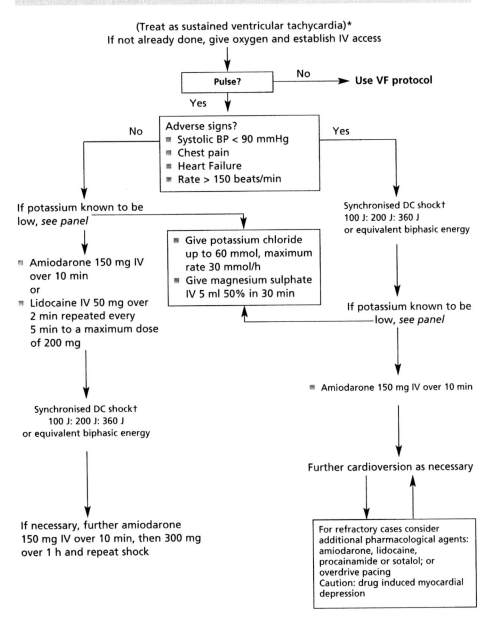

(Treat as sustained ventricular tachycardia)*
If not already done, give oxygen and establish IV access

Pulse? — No → **Use VF protocol**

Yes

Adverse signs?
■ Systolic BP < 90 mmHg
■ Chest pain
■ Heart Failure
■ Rate > 150 beats/min

No / Yes

If potassium known to be low, *see panel*

■ Amiodarone 150 mg IV over 10 min
or
■ Lidocaine IV 50 mg over 2 min repeated every 5 min to a maximum dose of 200 mg

■ Give potassium chloride up to 60 mmol, maximum rate 30 mmol/h
■ Give magnesium sulphate IV 5 ml 50% in 30 min

Synchronised DC shock†
100 J: 200 J: 360 J
or equivalent biphasic energy

If potassium known to be low, *see panel*

Synchronised DC shock†
100 J: 200 J: 360 J
or equivalent biphasic energy

Amiodarone 150 mg IV over 10 min

Further cardioversion as necessary

If necessary, further amiodarone 150 mg IV over 10 min, then 300 mg over 1 h and repeat shock

For refractory cases consider additional pharmacological agents: amiodarone, lidocaine, procainamide or sotalol; or overdrive pacing
Caution: drug induced myocardial depression

Doses throughout are based on an adult of average body weight.
*For paroxysms of tosades de pointes, use magnesium as above or overdrive pacing (expert help strongly recommended).
†DC shock is always given under sedation/general anaesthesia.

Answer – Self-test 8: Narrow Complex Tachycardia

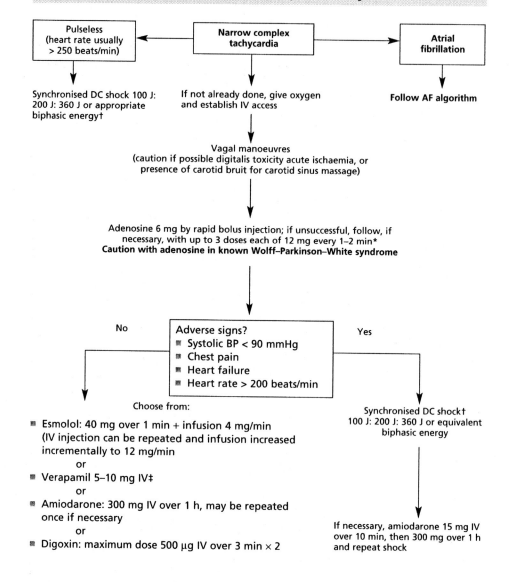

Doses throughout are based on an adult of average body weight.
A starting dose of 6 mg adenosine is currently outside the UK license for this agent.
*Theophylline and related compounds block the effect of adenosine. Patients on dipyridamole, carbamazepine, or with denervated hearts have a marked exaggerated effect which may be hazardous.
†DC shock is always given under sedation/general anaesthesia.
‡Not to be used in patients receiving beta-blockers.

Answer – Self-test 9: Newborn Life Support

Dry the baby; remove any wet cloth and cover

↓

Initial assessment at birth
Start the clock or note the time
Assess: COLOUR, TONE, BREATHING, HEART RATE

↓

If not breathing . . .

↓

Control the airway
Head in the neutral position

↓

Support the breathing
If not breathing – FIVE INFLATION BREATHS (each 2–3 s duration)
Confirm a response: increase in HEART RATE or visible CHEST MOVEMENT

↓

If there is no response
Double check head position and apply JAW THRUST
5 inflation breaths
Confirm a response: increase in HEART RATE or visible CHEST MOVEMENT

↓

If there is *still* no response
a) Use a second person (if available) to help with airway control and repeat inflation breaths
b) Inspect the oropharynx under direct vision (is suction needed?) and repeat inflation breaths
c) Insert an oropharyngeal (Guedel) airway and repeat inflation breaths
Consider intubation
Confirm a response: increase in HEART RATE or visible CHEST MOVEMENT

↓

When the chest is moving
Continue the ventilation breaths if no spontaneous breathing

↓

Check the heart rate
If the heart rate is not detectable *or slow* (less than around 60 bpm) and NOT increasing

↓

Start chest compressions
First confirm chest movement – if chest not moving return to airway
3 chest compressions to 1 breath for 30 s

↓

Reassess heart rate
If improving – stop chest compressions, continue ventilation if not breathing
If heart rate still slow, continue ventilation and chest compressions
Consider venous access and drugs at this stage

AT ALL STAGES, ASK. DO YOU NEED HELP?
In the presence of meconium remember: Screaming babies have an open airway.
Floppy babies: have a look.

ANAESTHETIC EQUIPMENT

5

Anaesthetic Equipment 1   *(Answers on page 173)*

Tracheal tube

Questions

1. A nasal tube has the same curvature as an oral tube.   True   False

2. A nasal tube can be identified by having a longer pilot tube.   True   False

3. Murphy's eye is to prevent one lung anaesthesia.   True   False

4. A reinforced tube will not kink.   True   False

5. The low pressure cuff is designed to only produce a complete seal during inspiration in positive pressure ventilation   True   False

6. A tube of larger internal diameter will have a greater resistance to spontaneous breathing than a narrow tube.   True   False

7. Resistance to flow in a tube is inversely related to viscosity.   True   False

8. The correct length for a tracheal tube is related to the distance from the tragus to the side of the mouth.   True   False

9. The diameter of the tube in children is given by 4mm or 4.5 mm + 1/4 age   True   False

10. A red rubber tube is more likely than a PVC tube to be ignited by a laser beam.   True   False

Anaesthetic Equipment 2 *(Answers on page 174)*

One lung anaesthesia

Write out a sequence for inserting the double lumen tube and inflating the cuffs.

Then check that one lung can be inflated independently of the other.

Use the labels on the diagram opposite to identify each step.

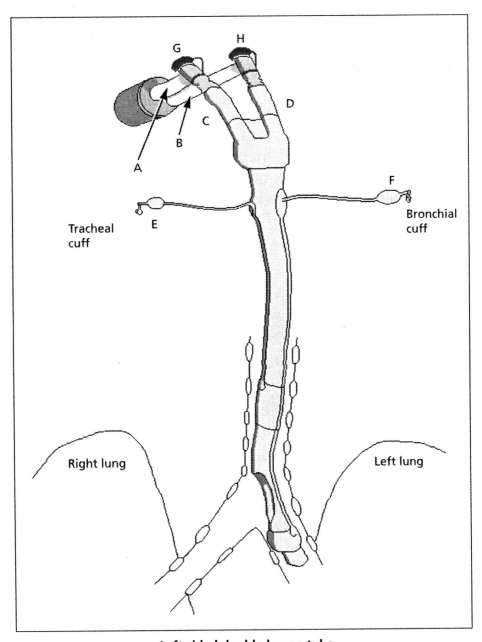

G

H

D

C

B

A

F

Bronchial cuff

Tracheal cuff

E

Right lung

Left lung

Left sided double lumen tube

Anaesthetic Equipment 3 *(Answers on page 175)*

Nuffield ventilator

A Bain circuit has been connected to a Nuffield ventilator for IPPV as shown. opposite. A fresh gas flow of 6 l/min is set.

Questions

1. The flow of anaesthetic gas that the patient receives from the anaesthetic machine will not be diluted by oxygen, or other driving gas, if the volume of the connecting tubing from the ventilator up to the patient is 500 ml.   True   False

2. The rate of ventilation will be 12 breaths per minute.   True   False

3. The I:E ratio is set at 1:2.   True   False

4. The tidal volume will be 1000 ml (1 litre).   True   False

5. The expired gas will be void to a scavenger at point A.   True   False

6. The connections at point C are 22 mm in diameter.   True   False

7. A fresh gas flow of 70 ml/kg/min and IPPV with the parameters set is likely to be associated with nomocapnoea in a normal adult.   True   False

8. The ventilator could be driven by compressed air without affecting the patient's oxygenation if the volume of the connecting tubing from the ventilator is adequate.   True   False

9. A spirometer at point D will not measure accurately the expired tidal volume.   True   False

10. The longer the tubing between points B and C the lower will be the minute ventilation.   True   False

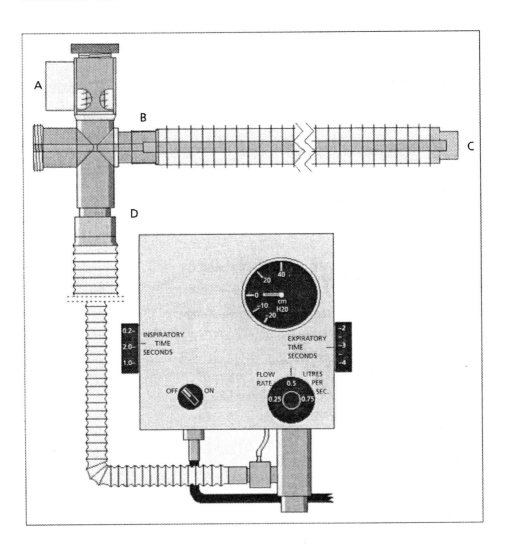

Anaesthetic Equipment 4   (Answers on page 176)

Laryngeal mask airway

Questions

1. What are the laryngeal mask sizes and forms that are available?

2. What does ST on the tube stand for?

3. What does a laryngeal mask consist of and what it is made from?

4. Is the laryngeal mask autoclavable?

5. How many times can the airway be safely cleaned and re-used?

6. What is the correct method for introducing the airway?

7. What does the distal end of the airway lodge against?

8. Does cricoid pressure prevent the correct placement of the airway?

9. How much air should be used in the size 3 airway?

10. Why is the airway associated with a higher PEEP than is present with a tracheal tube?

11. What tests and precautions should be performed before using the laryngeal mask airway?

12. Who developed this airway?

13. What are indications for using this airway?

14. What are the complications of using the airway?

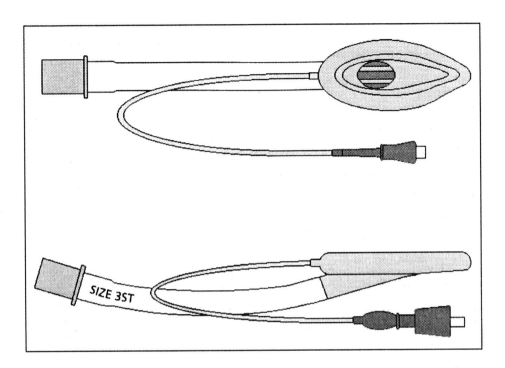

Anaesthetic Equipment 5 *(Answers on page 178)*

Bain Circuit

Questions

1. Which Mapleson breathing system does the Bain circuit best represent?

2. It is more suitable for use with children than a Mapleson A system?

3. The normal length is 1 meter. What happens if the length is increased?

4. What is the effect of a disconnection at C?

5. What are the standard sizes for the connections at A B and D?

6. What is the maximum pressure to open an APL valve before it is closed? What is the minimum pressure?

7. What limits the pressure and hence barotrauma to the lung?

8. What is the reservoir bag made from and what are its functions?

9. What reservoir bag sizes are available? What are the problems if the bag is too big or too small?

10. What is the volume of the breathing system?

11. What happens if the reservoir bag is removed?

12. What should the fresh gas flow (fgf) be to prevent rebreathing when breathing spontaneously?

13. What should the fresh gas flow be to prevent rebreathing for controlled ventilation?

14. What fresh gas flow can be used for normocapnia?

15. How would you check the integrity of the Bain Circuit?

16. Is this system suitable for use in a MRI scanner?

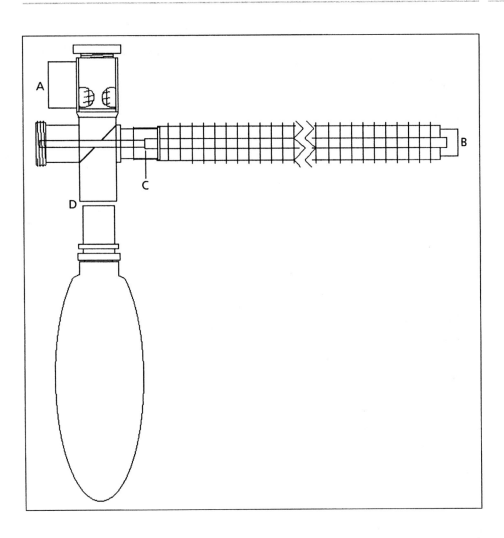

Anaesthetic Equipment 6

(Answers on page 180)

This vaporiser (diagram opposite):

1. Is suitable for draw over anaesthesia.   True   False

2. Is temperature compensated by means
   of an expanding bellows.   True   False

3. Can be used for halothane with no recalibration.   True   False

4. Would work more efficiently if it had a matt
   black finish.   True   False

5. With a splitting ratio of 9:1, the delivered vapour
   concentration would be approximately 3%.   True   False

6. Has a filling system allowing only isoflurane
   to be used.   True   False

7. Can work safely tilted up to 40 degrees.   True   False

8. On the back bar of the anaesthetic machine the
   vaporiser should be placed downstream of an
   enflurane vaporiser.   True   False

9. Will give a higher concentration than set, with
   a fresh gas flow rate of 15 l/min.   True   False

10. Can give up to 6.7 MAC isoflurane.   True   False

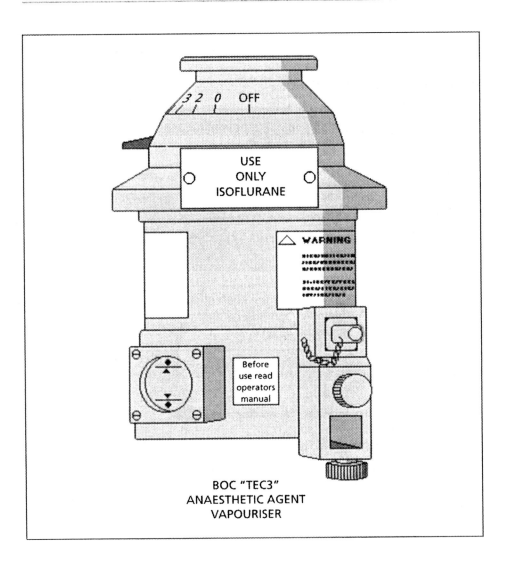

BOC "TEC3"
ANAESTHETIC AGENT
VAPOURISER

Anaesthetic Equipment 7 (Answers on page 181)

Boyle anaesthetic machine

Questions

You may be asked to demonstrate how you would perform a pre-anaesthetic check on the Boyle machine. You should practise this check regularly before coming to the examination. For a method you should refer to the booklet produced by the Association of Anaesthetists (AAGBI). In normal circumstances you will probably not find an error. In an examination, several faults may be made to the machine for you to demonstrate.

This is not a detailed check of the machine but some special points to note are:

The machine in the examination hall will not be connected to a wall pipeline supply so always start as if the machine were disconnnected from the wall supply. Turn on only the oxygen cylinder. Check the cylinder gauge, open the rotameter. Pressure test and look for a dip on the rotameter. No dip means a leak. Turn on the vaporiser and pressure test again. Mark 3 vaporisers will leak from the back bar without being turned on, Mark 4 must be turned on to check that the back bar seals are intact. Check that it is oxygen with an oxygen analyser.

Turn off the oxygen cylinder and with the rotameter open empty the oxygen from the circuits, the oxygen failure warning should sound. Turn on the nitrous oxide. Check the gauge, turn on the rotameter. No gas should flow if fitted with a modern oxygen failure device. Now turn on the oxygen cylinder, making sure that the oxygen rotameter is off, and the nitrous oxide may now flow on older machines. Turning the nitrous oxide rotameter on may also cause the oxygen to flow if the machine is fitted with a minimum oxygen concentration device which links the nitrous oxide to the oxygen.

Look at the breathing circuit and check the APL valve, connecting tubing and reservoir bag. Finally, check the scavenging and suction systems.

The diagram opposite shows a number of errors. List the errors that you see and explain what the correct position should be.

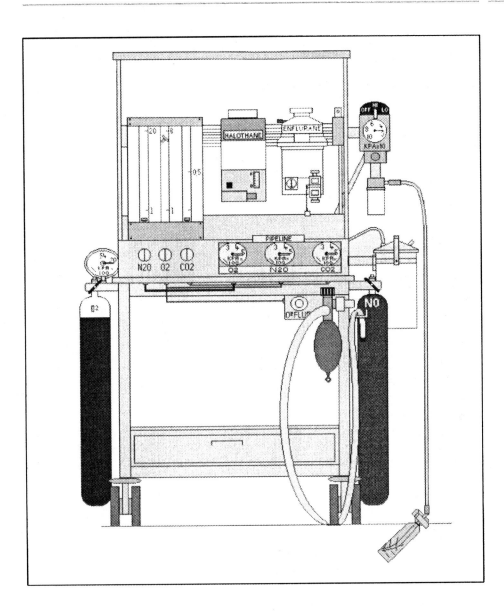

Anaesthetic Equipment 8   (Answers on page 182)

Now write out exactly the Association of Anaesthetists of Great Britain and Ireland checklist for Anaesthetic Apparatus. Write out each stage.

Anaesthetic Equipment 9   (Answers on page 185)

Circle breathing system

Questions

1. Label the parts of the circle illustrated on the diagram opposite.

2. Describe how to check the circle system.

3. What is the minimum fresh gas flow required in a circuit with the soda lime in the circuit?

4. What is the minimum fresh gas flow required in a circuit with the soda lime out of the circuit?

5. Which volatile agents react with soda lime?

6. Name some advantages of using a closed circuit with low flows.

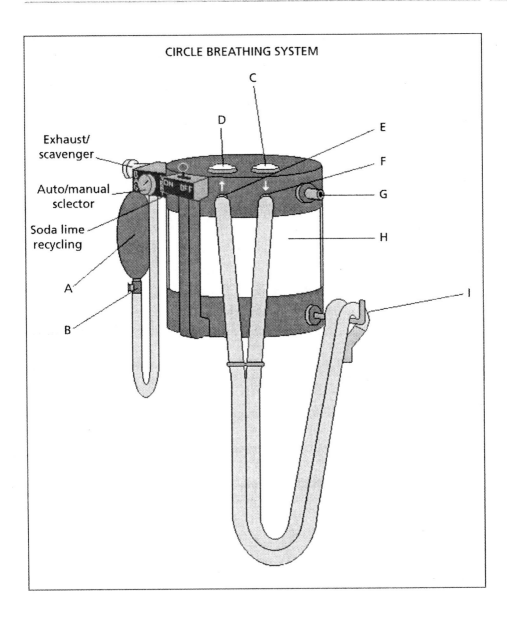

CIRCLE BREATHING SYSTEM

C

D

E

F

Exhaust/
scavenger

Auto/manual
sclector

ON OFF

G

Soda lime
recycling

H

A

I

B

Anaesthetic Equipment 10 *(Answers on page 187)*

Reducing valve

Questions

1. What is this apparatus used for?

2. What is **A** and what is the physical principle that underlies the working of **A**?

3. What is special about **B**?

4. What two ways are there for making the gas flow?

5. What happens when the patient breathes in with reference to **C**?

6. What instructions should the patient receive in order to use this apparatus?

7. What additional information should the labouring patient receive?

8. What is Entonox and what is peculiar about it?

9. How would you recognise an Entonox cylinder?

10. When would it be unwise to use Entonox for pain relief?

11. Why should this apparatus only be used for self-administration?

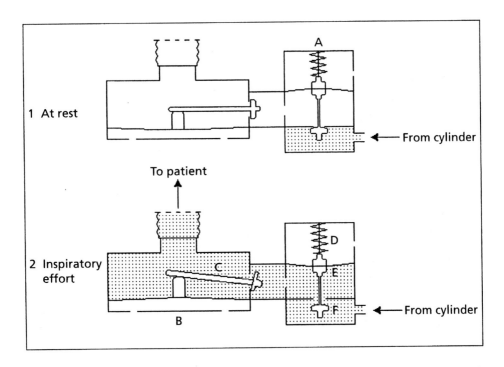

1 At rest

To patient

2 Inspiratory
effort

A

From cylinder

B

C

D

E

F

From cylinder

Anaesthetic Equipment 11 *(Answers on page 188)*

Questions

1. What is this apparatus?

2. How does it work?

3. What is the physical principle which allows it to work?

4. What is the minimum oxygen flow that should be used?

5. What will happen if the oxygen flow is set low?

6. What advantages does this mask have over a variable performance mask?

7. Name one other piece of apparatus that uses the same principle.

8. How is it possible to give 100% oxygen with a facemask?

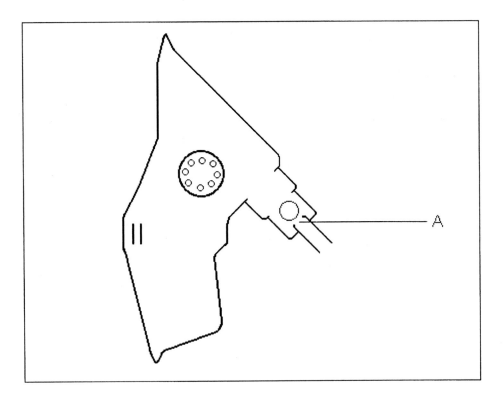

Anaesthetic Equipment 12 *(Answers on page 189)*

Questions

1. What is the name of this apparatus?

2. What can it be used for?

3. What is shape of the cross-section at **A** and at **B**?

4. Why does the scale move from 1 to 2 when a cylinder is attached to **C** and the pressure increased to **D**?

5. What units might be used for the scale?

6. What is the pressure if a full cylinder of: (a) oxygen, (b) nitrous oxide (c) carbon dioxide, (d) Entonox, is attached?

7. What will affect the pressure in a cylinder?

8. What are the gas laws?

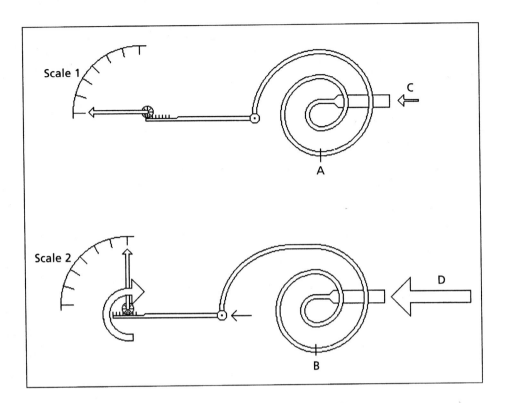

Answers
Anaesthetic Equipment

Answers – Anaesthetic Equipment 1

1. **False** – The nasal tube is the arc of a larger circle than an oral tube.

2. **False** – The pilot tube is the same length but is attached to a greater length of the wall of the tube.

3. **False** – Murphy's eye is to reduce the incidence of obstruction of the terminal opening. It may also help to prevent obstruction of the right upper lobe bronchus when it comes off at the carina or from the trachea.

4. **False** – Reinforced tubes can kink, particularly if the connector does not enter the reinforced part of the tube.

5. **True** – The seal is dynamic, produced by the back pressure of air in the trachea.

6. **False** – The larger the diameter the lower the resistance.

7. **False** – Resistance is directly proportional to viscosity in laminar flow and to density in turbulent flow.

8. **True** – In adults the length is x 1½ this distance. In children it is × 2 this distance.

9. **True**.

10. **False** – PVC ignites quicker.

Answer – Anaesthetic Equipment 2

1. Intubate the trachea using a fibre-optic laryngoscope or until the tube will go no further.

2. Inflate the tracheal cuff E.

3. Note the inflation pressure and tidal volume. Check for equal entry of air into both lungs.

To ensure left lung ventilation.

4. Clamp at the connector A

5. Release stopper at G.

6. Inflate and listen for leak from C.

7. Inflate bronchial cuff F until leak stops. The presence of a leak can also be assessed by comparing inspiratory and expiratory volumes and by detecting carbon dioxide with a capnograph at G. A measure of expired volume is useful to ensure that the same tidal/minute volume is achieved with one lung as with two lungs and that carbon dioxide is being eliminated. Measure the oxygen saturation.

8. Release clamp at A and stopper G.

Ensure right lung ventilation.

9. Clamp at B.

10. Open stopper at H.

11. Inflate and listen for a leak if bronchial or tracheal cuffs are not adequately inflated.

    Measure the volume expired and pressure for inflation to ensure that they are within the physiological range.

    Depending on which lung is to be ventilated the tidal volume may have to be adjusted to keep the inspiratory pressure within the normal range.

    Measure the oxygen saturation.

12. Stopper H and release clamp at B.

13. The best way of checking the position of the tube is to use a fibre-optic bronchoscope.

Answers – Anaesthetic Equipment 3

1. **False** – The ventilator is set to deliver 1000 ml per breath. Mixing will be prevented, in this example, if the volume of the tubing between the ventilator and the patient is 1 litre or over.

2. **True** – 2 seconds in, 3 seconds out – 5 seconds per breath.

3. **False** – I:E ratio is 2:3.

4. **False** – The tidal volume will be 2 seconds inspiration at 0.5 l/s which equals 1 litre plus the fresh gas flow in 2 seconds. If the fresh gas flow is 6 1/min this will be 100 ml in 1 second and 200 ml in 2 seconds. Tidal volume will be 1200 ml.

5. **False** – At the bottom of the expiratory valve on the ventilator. The valve at A should be shut.

6. **True.**

7. **True.**

8. **True** – The ventilator driving gas will not reach the patient if the volume of the connecting tubing and the expiratory part of the co-axial tubing is greater than the tidal volume.

9. **True** – As fresh gas flow may increase the volume measured.

10. **True** – As the ventilator will waste some of the gas in expanding/ventilating the tubing.

Answers – Anaesthetic Equipment 4

1. New sizes are being introduced. The ordinary sizes are: 1, 2, 2½, 3, 3ST, 4, 5. There are reinforced, intubating and MRI laryngeal mask airways.

2. ST stands for short.

3. Consists of:
   a. Tube – transparent. Large internal diameter to reduce the work of breathing. Size 3–9 mm; size 4–10 mm. The proximal end has a standard 15 mm connection.
   b. Elliptical cuff designed to form a relatively air tight seal around the posterior perimeter of the larynx. It is permeable to air, nitrous oxide and other gases.
   c. Pilot balloon with self-sealing valve. A non-metallic valve is available for use in MRI.
   d. Slits at junction of tube and cuff to prevent epiglottis from obstructing the laryngeal mask. Obstruction still occurs in up to 10% of patients.

   Made from silicon rubber not plastic. Care in patients with latex allergy.

4. Autoclavable at 134–139°C or washed and cleaned in detergent.

5. The manufacturer recommends 40 uses; i.e. 39 re-uses.

6. Three hands are needed: one to hold the laryngeal mask airway, one to flex the neck and one to draw the jaw forward. The cuff is inflated back on itself, lubricated on the palatal side. Inserted through the mouth passing against the palate. It is recommended that the tube be held in the fashion of holding a pencil with the index finger along the tube.

7. The inferior constrictor.

8. Yes. The distal end of the airway lies between the cricoid and the body of C6.

9. Size 1–4 ml, size 2–10 ml, size 3–20 ml, size 4–30 ml, size 5–40 ml.

10. The adductors of the cords contract during normal expiration thus producing a small PEEP. The tracheal tube prevents this adduction and so eliminates a natural PEEP.

11. Inspect the lumen – patent, the cuff inflation, the slits intact. It should be possible to bend the tube through 180° without kinking. Ensure that the patient is not likely to regurgitate.

12. Archie Brain.

13. Indications include:
    - Use instead of a face mask.
    - Effective to maintain airway in spontaneously breathing patient.
    - Effective for IPPV and will maintain some PEEP.
    - Difficult airway.
    - Aid to intubation with a bougie or narrow lumen tracheal tube. Use airway without slits.

14. Complications:

- Does not protect against inspiration.
- Despite the slits about 10% of patients develop airway obstruction due to down folding of the epiglottis.
- Only usable 40 times.
- Complete rotation may result in airway obstruction.

Answers – Anaesthetic Equipment 5

1. Mapleson D. You must know the Mapleson classification.

2. Yes. Because the apparatus dead space is limited to the space from the fresh gas inlet to the patient. It can also be considered as a T piece with a reservoir bag and an adjustable pressure limiting (APL) valve.

3. Increasing the length will slightly increase the resistance to expiration.

4. A disconnection at C means that the whole of the outer tubing becomes apparatus dead space

5. Connections are: A 30 mm for scavenging, B internal 15 mm to the tracheal tube, B external 22 mm to one way valve or breathing system, D 22 mm to breathing system.

6. The maximum pressure is 60 cm H_2O. Minimum pressure about 2 cm H_2O and even less with the spring removed, but the valve must then be used in a vertical position.

7. The elasticity of the reservoir bag.

8. The reservoir bag is made of plastic or anti-static rubber. Its functions include: a reservoir for inspiratory gases, a limit to barotrauma to the lung, an indicator of respiration, mixes the gases, manual ventilation.

9. Bags are available in 500 ml, 1, 2 and 5 litres. Too small and it may not store sufficient gas for inspiration, too big and it fails to move with respiration. Normally the bag is 2 litres for adults.

10. 1 meter long × 22 mm internal diameter = 400 ml/meter.

11. Air may be inspired but only if the fresh gas flow is less than 20–30 l/min for an adult.

12. To prevent rebreathing totally, the fgf should be equal to the peak inspiratory flow rate of about 30 l/min. Mapleson calculated a theoretical value for normocapnia of 2–2.5 × minute ventilation or 15 litres for an adult.

13. The same as for spontaneously breathing.

14. 70–80 ml/kg/min breathing spontaneously and 100 ml/kg/min for controlled ventilation.

15. *a.* Visual inspection, correct configuration, no kinks, no obstruction, no foreign bodies.

    All connections securely fastened by twisting and pulling.

    APL valve opens and closes.

    b. Occlusion test: set oxygen at 6 l/min close the APL valve, occlude the inner tube at the patient outlet. Observe a drop in the bobbin, valve on back bar may open, reservoir bag should not inflate.

c. APL valve closed. Fill reservoir bag, open oxygen flush and reservoir bag should collapse due to a venturi effect of the flow of oxygen on the gas in the outer tube.

A similar effect is generated by temporary occluding the gas outlet and then letting go.

16. Yes. Providing the plastic tubing is long enough that all the metal parts are outside the magnetic field.

Answers – Anaesthetic Equipment 6

1. **False** – The internal resistance is too great, causing an unacceptable increase in the work of breathing when used for spontaneous respiration.

2. **False** – TEC vaporisers use a bimetallic strip. Penlon, Drager and EMO use expanding bellows.

3. **True** – The calibration of a vaporiser depends on the saturated vapour pressure (SVP) of the agent. At 20°C, halothane and isoflurane have near identical SVP (32 and 33 kPa respectively).

4. **True** – A matt black finish would increase absorption of heat from the environment, reducing temperature drop during vaporisation.

5. **True** – Isoflurane's SVP is 33 kPa, so assuming close to 100% efficiency of vaporisation, passing all the fresh gas flow through the vaporising chamber would give: $33 \times 100/101 = 32.6\%$. With a splitting ratio of 9 to 1, 9 litres bypass the chamber while 1 litre passes through it. Therefore the vapour is diluted by a factor of $(9 + 1)$, and the final vapour concentration is 3.26%.

6. **True** – The Fraser Sweatman valve is used to connect the isoflurane bottle to the vaporiser. Its design is such that it will only fit on to an isoflurane bottle and an isoflurane vaporiser. Some TEC 3s do not have this filling system but all TEC 4s do.

7. **False** – When tilted more than 30 degrees, liquid isoflurane can pass into the bypass tube, resulting in a high delivered concentration. The later model TEC vaporisers are designed so this cannot happen.

8. **True** – In the event of both vaporisers being turned on, isoflurane could get into the enflurane vaporiser if that were downstream. On subsequent use, the higher potency and higher saturated vapour pressure of isoflurane could lead to an overdose being administered.

9. **False** – It will give a lower concentration due to incomplete saturation of the carrier gas at high flow rates.

10. **False** – It will give $5/1.15 = 4.3$ MAC.

Answers – Anaesthetic Equipment 7

Test for oxygen first.

The mistakes are:

1. The oxygen cylinder has the wrong pressure gauge attached.

2. There is no cylinder spanner.

3. The oxygen rotameter column is normally at the left hand end as Boyle was left-handed, can be on the right, but never in the middle.

4. The central rotameter is displaced.

   The calibration on the rotameter column is wrong if the oxygen at 8 l is compared with the nitrous oxide at 20 litres. The two columns are usually calibrated to show almost the same flow rates at the top of the oxygen and nitrous oxide column.

5. The pipelines to the rotameter are linked to the wrong gauge reading and should show 4 kPa × 100 and no more.

6. CO_2 would not be on pipeline.

7. Nitrous oxide is not NO as on the cylinder.

8. There is no pressure gauge on the nitrous oxide cylinder.

9. The suction catheter is on the floor.

10. The suction pressure is at 3 kPa × 10 and should be at least 55 kPa when set on "High", particularly as someone has wrongly put a filter on the end and the bag will cause occlusion to sucking in air.

11. The suction tubing should enter the collecting reservoir not the filter chamber.

12. The breathing system is trapped under the wheel of the trolley.

13. There is no scavenging tubing attached to the APL valve.

14. Vaporisers in series that are not protected by an interlocking system and can be turned on together. The vaporiser that takes the most fresh gas flow should be nearest to the rotameters. This is the vaporiser with the lowest SVP and highest boiling point. With the downstream vaporiser having a higher SVP it will take in less fresh gas and so less contamination will occur. In this case enflurane (boiling point 56°C) should be next to the rotameter and halothane (boiling point 50°C) downstream.

15. The Mark III enflurane vaporiser has the filler port left open.

Answers – Anaesthetic Equipment 8

Stage 1. Check that the anaesthetic machine is connected to the electricity supply (if appropriate) and switched on. Take note of any information or labelling on the anaesthetic machine referring to the current status of the machine. Particular attention should be paid to recent servicing. Servicing labels should be fixed in the service logbook.

Stage 2. Check that an oxygen analyser is present on the anaesthetic machine. Ensure that the analyser is switched on, checked and calibrated.

Q. How do you calibrate the oxygen analyser?
A. Expose it to 100% oxygen and 21% oxygen of room air.

Q. Where should the oxygen analyser be placed?
A. The oxygen sensor should be placed where it can monitor the composition of the gases leaving the common gas outlet.

Stage 3. Identify and take note of the gases which are being supplied by pipeline, confirming with a "tug-test" that each pipeline is correctly inserted into the appropriate gas supply terminal.

Carbon dioxide cylinders should not be present on the anaesthetic machine unless requested by the anaesthetist.

Q. What should be applied to an empty yoke and why?
A. A blanking plug should be fitted to any empty cylinder yoke as the reducing valve is not a one-way valve and gas from one cylinder can leak back.

Q. What stops leaks between cylinder and yoke?
A. A Bodok valve – **B**ritish **O**xygen **Dock**ing device (when BOC supplied all cylinders).

- Check that the anaesthetic machine is connected to a supply of oxygen and that an adequate supply of oxygen is available from a reserve oxygen cylinder.
- Check that adequate supplies of other gases (nitrous oxide, air) are available and connected as appropriate.
- Check that all pipeline pressure gauges in use on the anaesthetic machine indicate 400 kPa.

Stage 4. Check the operation of flowmeters.

- Ensure that each flow control valve operates smoothly and that the bobbin moves freely throughout its range.
- Check the operation of the emergency oxygen bypass control.

Stage 5. Check the vaporiser(s):

- Ensure that each vaporiser is adequately but not over filled.
- Ensure that each vaporiser is correctly seated on the back bar and not tilted.
- Check the vaporiser for leaks (**with vaporiser on and off**) by temporarily occluding the common gas outlet.

Q. Which vaporisers can leak from the selectatec backbar connection when turned off and which leak when turned on?
A. Mark 3 leak turned off and Mark 4 leak only when turned on.

Q. What should happen when the common gas outlet is occluded?
A. With a flow of 6 l/min the rotameter float should drop about 0.5 cm. If the obstruction persists the relief valve on the backbar will open at about 40 kPa

When checks have been completed turn the vaporiser(s) off.

A leak test should be performed immediately after changing any vaporiser.

Stage 6. Check the breathing system.

- The system should be visually inspected for correct configuration. All connections should be secured by "push and twist".
- A pressure leak test should be performed on the breathing system by occluding the patient port and compressing the reservoir bag.
- The correct operation of unidirectional valves should be carefully checked.

Stage 7. Check that the ventilator is configured appropriately for its intended use.

- Ensure that the ventilator tubing is correctly configured and securely attached.
- Set the controls for use and ensure that an adequate pressure is generated during the inspiratory phase.
- Check that the pressure relief valve functions.
- Check that the disconnect alarm functions correctly.
- Ensure that an alternative means to ventilate the patient's lungs is available.

Q. What alternative means should be available?
A. A self-inflating bag and mask. Check how to dismantle and reassemble a self-inflating bag and valve.

Q. There are two types of Ambu one-way valve, how do they differ?
A. One valve has two diaphragms in it. This means that gas flow is one-way into the patient and then expelled through the other arm of the T. No air can be entrained if the patient breathes spontaneously. Suitable for giving a GA. The second type only has one diaphragm. Air is forced into the patient and cannot return into the bag. If the patient breathes spontaneously they can breath in air. Suitable for resuscitation.

Stage 8. Check that the anaesthetic gas scavenging system is switched on and is functioning correctly.

- Ensure that the tubing is attached to the appropriate expiratory port(s) of the breathing system or ventilator.

Stage 9. Check that all ancillary equipment, which may be needed, is present and working.

- This includes laryngoscopes, intubation aids, intubation forceps, bougies etc, and appropriately sized facemasks, airways, tracheal tubes and connectors.
- Check that the suction apparatus is functioning and that all connections are secure.
- Check that the patient can be tilted head-down on the trolley, operating table or bed.

Stage 10. Ensure that the appropriate monitoring equipment is present, switched on and calibrated ready for use.

- Set all default alarm limits as appropriate.

(It may be necessary to place the monitors in the stand-by mode to avoid unnecessary alarms before being connected to the patient.)

The checklist for Anaesthetic Apparatus is reproduced by kind permission of The Association of Anaesthetists of Great Britain and Ireland.

Answers – Anaesthetic Equipment 9

1. a. 2 litre reservoir bag.
   b. APL valve
   c. Inspiratory valve
   d. Expiratory valve
   e. Expiratory port
   f. Inspiratory port
   g. Port for fresh gas
   h. Soda lime canister
   i. Y patient connection.

2. Check that each part is attached: The connection to the gas outlet from the Boyle machine. Soda lime canister attached. Circle tubing with Y connector to patient. Reservoir bag attached; APL pressure relief valve (check if two valves are present) and scavenging port.

To test for a leak in the circuit: Attach a reservoir bag to the Y patient connector. Fill the circuit with gas to a pressure of 40 mmHg. If the reservoir bag is older, a pressure of 30 mmHg may be the most that can be reached. This pressure should be held for at least 5 minutes.

To test whether the valves are competent attach a reservoir bag on the patient Y connection. Detach the inspiratory limb from the block to which the soda lime is attached. Hold the palm of the hand against the outlet from the canister block. No gas should flow backwards to come out of the inspiratory tubing coming from the patient Y connection. Reconnect. Alternatively, take the expiratory limb off the canister block and put the palm of the hand over the expiratory limb of the circuit coming from the patient. No gas should come from the expiratory outlet of the canister block.

3. There are two answers depending on whether oxygen alone is used or whether a second gas such as nitrous oxide is used. The oxygen requirement of the patient will be 250–400 ml/min depending on the rate of metabolism. If 100% oxygen is used, once the circuit is filled this basal flow should be supplemented so that nitrogen, carbon monoxide and some trace gases do not accumulate.

If there is nitrous oxide and oxygen in the circle then the oxygen concentration in the circuit is given by: oxygen in minus oxygen used, divided by total gas in minus oxygen used. Flows of 500 ml of oxygen and 500 ml of nitrous oxide with 250 ml oxygen used will give an oxygen concentration of 250 ml/750 ml or 33%. At these flows the oxygen in the circuit must be monitored.

$$O_2\% \text{ in circuit} = \frac{O_2 \text{ in} - O_2 \text{ used}}{\text{Total gas in} - O_2 \text{ used}}$$

4. Without carbon dioxide absorption the elimination of carbon dioxide depends on the amount of gas escaping through the expiratory valve and the nature of that gas. If the circuit can be arranged to preferentially retain the dead space gas and dump the alveolar gas, without dumping fresh gas, then a fresh gas flow equal to or just above alveolar ventilation may be sufficient. If dead space gas is dumped in preference to fresh gas then higher flows are needed equivalent to minute ventilation. If fresh gas and dead space gases are dumped in preference to alveolar gas then flows of up to twice the minute ventilation will be required. The fresh gas flow depends on the relative positions of the reservoir bag, the APL valve, and the IN port for the fresh gas.

5. Virtually all volatile agents react with soda lime including: trichloroethylene, sevoflurane and halothane. It is important clinically if the products are toxic as with trichloroethylene, or are produced in large quantities and so alter the total composition of the gas in the circle as with sevoflurane.

6. *a.* Reduces pollution
   b. Reduces cost
   c. Conserves heat
   d. Conserves water vapour (not useful if using an HMEF).

Answers – Anaesthetic Equipment 10

1. The self-administration of Entonox.

2. **A** is a reducing valve. A high pressure is applied to a small area **F** and this is equated with a lower pressure over a large area **E**. The force or energy of the gas remains constant. At the same time a spring **D** ensures that as the high cylinder pressure falls the reduced lower pressure remains constant by making the opening into the chamber larger.

3. It is a flexible diaphragm.

4. The negative pressure of inspiration, and hand pressure on the diaphragm **B** used to test the apparatus.

5. The negative pressure draws the diaphragm up and displaces the bar **C**. This opens the aperture and the pressure drops in the chamber of the reducing valve. The reduced pressure then causes the valve to open and gas flows from the cylinder at high rates.

6. Keep the mask with an air tight seal to the face (or a mouthpiece). Draw a deep inspiration, through the one-way valve on the mask and breathe out through the mask.

7. In labour try to predict the next contraction and start breathing the Entonox before the contraction starts.

8. Entonox is a 50:50 mixture of oxygen and nitrous oxide. The oxygen reduces the critical temperature of oxygen to minus 7°C.

9. The cylinder is blue with a blue and white colour. It has a single pin on the yoke.

10. When nitrous oxide would expand into a cavity such as in a pneumothorax or bowel obstruction.

11. Self-administration makes it safe. If the patient loses consciousness or vomits they will not maintain an airtight seal. They will lay the mask aside and stop taking more nitrous oxide until they regain awareness.

Answers – Anaesthetic Equipment 11

1. A fixed performance oxygen mask.

2. Oxygen flows through the orifice **A** and entrains air before the gas mixture passes into the facemask.

3. The Bernoulli effect. The flow of oxygen speeds up as it passes through the orifice at the end of the delivery tube. As the kinetic energy increases there is a loss of potential energy. The total energy stays the same. Hence the pressure above the orifice drops. It is devised so that the drop in pressure becomes a negative pressure and so air is entrained. The tube above this is for mixing of the gases.

4. The minimum flow is stamped on each mask and varies with the fixed concentration delivered. The flow must deliver at least the peak inspiratory flow rate for the patient so that no air is drawn into the mask during inspiration. This is about 35 l/min for an adult.

5. If the oxygen is set too low the patient will drawn air into the mask during inspiration and dilute the oxygen concentration coming into the mask. The amount of air entrained at the venturi will be proportionally less. The ratio of air to oxygen remains the same at the venturi and this fixed concentration will be delivered into the mask.

6. Used correctly it delivers a known fixed oxygen concentration.

7. Suction devices, particularly for portable use and powered by a gas cylinder. Oxygen blenders.

8. To deliver 100% oxygen, two types of mask can be used. A variable performance mask with the peak inspiratory flow of oxygen 30 to 40 l/min. A mask with a reservoir bag attached and a one-way valve. Oxygen is delivered into the bag. The patient breathes in from the bag and out to air. The Edinburgh mask achieves this with flows equal to the minute ventilation by breathing in from a reservoir bag and out through a one way valve.

Answers – Anaesthetic Equipment 12

1. A Bourdon gauge.

2. Measurement of pressure and also temperature.

3. The cross-section is **A** round, **B** an elliptical ovoid shape, like a rugby ball.

4. The tubing unwinds as the elliptical tubing expands and is made more circular.

5. PSI (pounds per square inch), kPa, atmospheres.

6. *a.* oxygen 1980 psi, 136 × 100 kPa, 134 atmospheres.
   b. nitrous oxide 639 psi, 44 × 100 kPa, 43 atmospheres.
   c. carbon dioxide 723 psi, 50 × 100 kPa, 49 atmospheres.
   d. Entonox 1980 psi, 136 × 100 kPa , 134 atmospheres.

7. The ambient temperature, the weight of gas in the cylinder, the critical temperature of the gas.

8. For a fixed mass of gas:

Boyle's Law: P is proportional to V (T constant)

Charle's Law: V is proportional to T (P constant)

Daltons $P = p1 + p2 + p3$

Avagadro's hypothesis. 1 gram molecule of a gas occupies 22.4 litres at STP.

MONITORING EQUIPMENT

6

Monitoring Equipment 1   *(Answers on page 201)*

Questions

1. A stethoscope has a diaphragm and a bell. What are they used for? What types of stethoscope are there?

2. Where should a stethoscope be placed after intubation?

3. Which patients are at risk from air embolism?

4. What are the signs of air embolism?

5. What treatment should be given if air embolism occurs?

Monitoring Equipment 2   *(Answers on page 203)*

Capnograph
Study the trace opposite.

Questions

1. The respiratory rate is 12 per minute.   True   False

2. The inspiratory: expiratory ratio is 1:1.   True   False

3. The slope BC is due to different alveolar time constants.   True   False

4. Inspiration ends at point C.   True   False

5. Expiration may start at point A.   True   False

6. The end tidal carbon dioxide shown will be the same
   as arterial carbon dioxide tension.   True   False

7. It could be obtained from an adult ventilated on a
   Bain circuit with a fresh gas flow of 8 l/min.   True   False

8. The capnograph works by absorption of infrared
   radiation at a wavelength of 4.3 μm   True   False

9. The presence of nitrous oxide will give a falsely low
   reading unless compensation is made.   True   False

10. Possible causes of the change seen after point X are:
    a. drop in cardiac output.   True   False
    b. partial disconnection of breathing system.   True   False

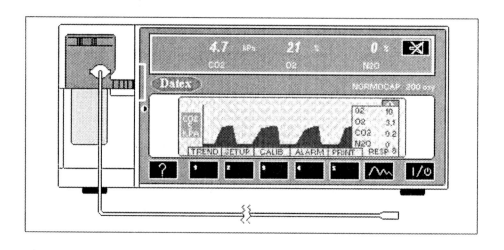

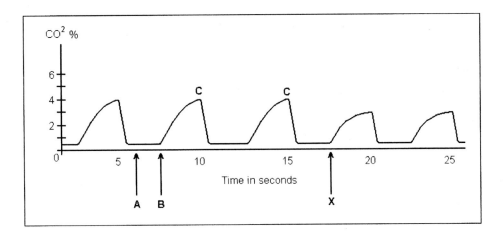

Monitoring Equipment 3 *(Answers on page 204)*

Traces

Questions

1. On the capnograph trace (below), label the beginning of expiration and the end of expiration, and the phases I, II, III, IV.

2. What can be learnt from the phase II slope?

3. What is the character of the phase III part of the curve?

4. What is the significance of the point E.

5. What factors affect the end tidal carbon dioxide concentration?

6. What happens in phase IV?

7. What can be learnt from trace A, B and C?

8. The site of CO_2 sampling diagram illustrates one point for sampling carbon dioxide. Is this the best place and what other precautions should be taken?

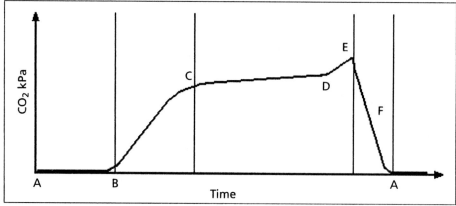

Capnograph waveform

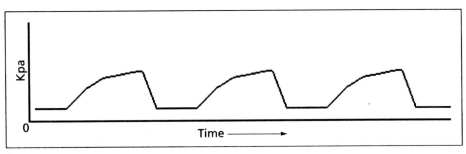

A

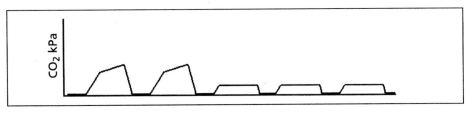

B

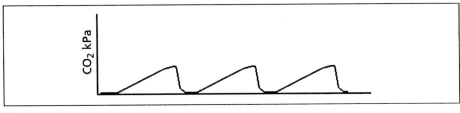

C

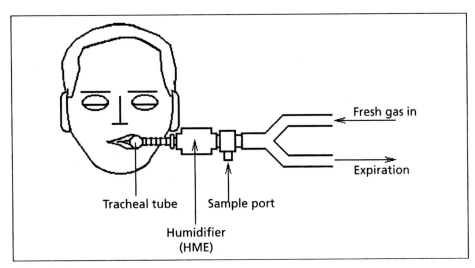

Site of CO_2 sampling

Monitoring Equipment 4 *(Answers on page 206)*

Questions

1. What means are available for measuring gas flow?

2. How can gas volumes be measured?

3. What is the device shown in the top figure and what does it measure?

4. What does it consist of and how does it work?

5. When is it less accurate and why?

6. Where should it be placed in the breathing system and why?

7. Why is it less accurate with time?

8. What is the device shown in the bottom figure?

9. How does it differ from the respirometer?

10. What does a Pneumotacograph measure?

11. How does it work?

12. What are the limits on the use of a Pneumotacograph?

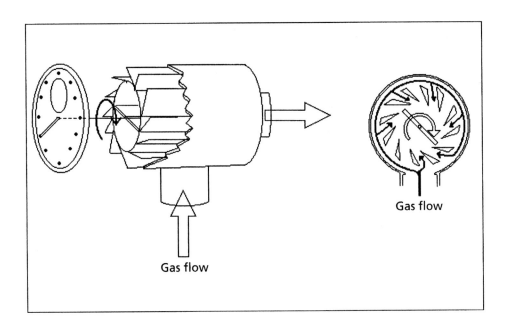

Gas flow

Gas flow

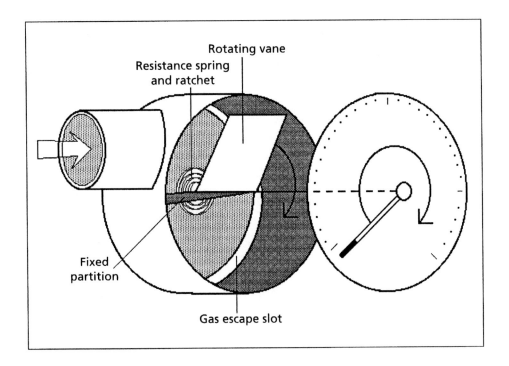

Rotating vane

Resistance spring
and ratchet

Fixed
partition

Gas escape slot

Monitoring Equipment 5 *(Answers on page 208)*

This apparatus:

Questions

1. Directly measures the oxygen saturation of haemoglobin. True False

2. Uses three wavelengths in the red and infra-red spectrum. True False

3. Gives an instant reading of oxygen saturation. True False

4. In heavy smokers, the reading will tend to be an overestimate of oxygen saturation. True False

5. A change in plasma hydrogen ion concentration from 40 to 28nm/l will increase haemloglobin affinity for oxygen. True False

6. Can be used reliably in the presence of a low pulse pressure. True False

7. In the jaundiced patient, the reading will be low. True False

8. The alarm level should be set at 85% in a healthy patient. True False

9. Can cause burns. True False

10. Is useful in assessing the severity of cyanide poisoning. True False

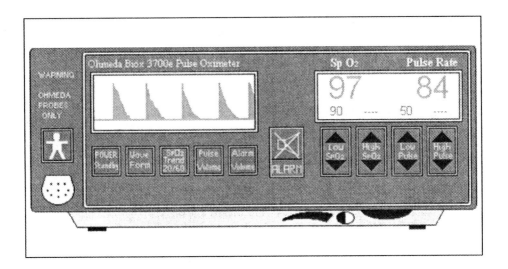

Answers
Monitoring Equipment

Answers – Monitoring equipment 1

1. Precordial. Diaphragm for high frequency sounds, bell for low frequency sounds

   Oesophageal stethoscope, particularly used in children.

2. *Uses*
   Pre-operative examination.

   Children can be monitored from induction to recovery by attaching a stethoscope to the left of the sternum. This will allow continuous monitoring of heart rate, respiration and particularly left-sided air entry to exclude right bronchial intubation. Detection of tracheal intubation and air embolism.

3. Check in axillae for air entry and over the stomach to exclude air entry. Fix to precordium to monitor for air embolism in patients at risk. (Better to fix a Doppler probe over the arch of the aorta.) Less than 1 ml of air IV will give a mill wheel murmur. Over 10 ml is necessary to reduce the cardiac output.

   Oesophageal stethoscope should be behind the heart in the lower third of the oesophagus. The cardia lies at 40 cm from the lips so the stethoscope should be 30–40 cm from the lips.

4. All patients. Air embolism occurs when air is sucked in through open veins or at cardiac surgery into the open heart. Whenever a vessel is opened by a catheter. Air can be drawn in through a CVP catheter, shunts for dialysis and cardiac by-pass pumps. Whenever a pump is used more air can be pumped in if the fluid reservoir becomes empty.

   Head and neck operations particularly when the head is raised above the heart level.

5. ▪ Sudden drop in cardiac output seen as fall in BP, rise in heart rate. Also, bronchospasm and pulmonary oedema.
   ▪ Drop in oxygen saturation, cyanosis.
   ▪ Reduced expired carbon dioxide concentration.

6. ▪ 100% oxygen – for resuscitation and will displace nitrogen from the air. Hyperbaric oxygen if easily available.
   ▪ Resuscitation ABC as for cardiac arrest.
   ▪ Flood the surgical area with saline and apply pressure through swabs.
   ▪ Raise venous pressure by head down tilt or pressure around the lower neck.

- Aspiration from the right ventricle can be attempted through a CVP catheter or if the chest is open directly from the heart.
- The patient should be turned onto their left side so that the right heart is upper most.
- The reduced cardiac output is as much due to frothing in the ventricle as to air in the circulation.

Answers – Monitoring Equipment 2

1. True.

2. False – It is impossible to tell the I:E ratio from this trace.

3. True – This is characteristic of a tracing with obstructive lung disease.

4. False – Expiration would end at point C.

5. True – Segment AB represents dead space gas.

6. False – As the CO_2 on the trace is still increasing at point C, end tidal CO_2 is unlikely to equal P_aCO_2 because of dilution with dead space gas.

7. True – The inspiratory CO_2 concentration does not return to zero. This rebreathing is compatible with the use of a Bain circuit at the stated fresh gas flow.

8. True.

9. False – It will give a higher reading. The absorption wavelength of infra-red radiation by nitrous oxide overlaps that of CO_2 causing over-reading.

10. a. True – Low cardiac output leads to reduced perfusion of some alveoli, increasing dead space, and a reduction in end tidal (but an increase in arterial) PCO_2.

    b. **True** – Due to dilution by room air.

Answers – Monitoring Equipment 3

1. This is a normal trace. A1 marks the end of expiration. Inspiration starts at A1 and continues to a point A2 halfway between A1 and B. The first part of expiration is anatomical dead space gas that is free of carbon dioxide from A2 to B. At B the anatomical dead space gas ends. Phase I – A2 to B, phase II – B to C, phase III – C to E, phase IV – A1 to A2.

2. Normal slope rise is rapid and almost vertical. A mixture of gas from the anatomical dead space and alveolar gas. The slope is determined by the different alveolar time constants. A more gradual slope indicates that the alveoli are receiving differing amounts of carbon dioxide due to perfusion mis-matches with ventilation. Or alveoli with different characteristics are emptying at different rates.

3. Phase III. This expiratory plateau is nearly horizontal. It rises slowly due to the effect of alveoli gas mixing with and being diluted by dead space gas at the beginning of expiration leading to gas coming entirely from alveoli at the end. The area under the curve is used to estimate cardiac output. The slope can also be used since MV CO_2 contributes to the generation of the slope.

4. E represents the end point of the plateau, called the end tidal carbon dioxide. This figure is normally 0.2–0.4 kPa (2–3 mmHg) lower than arterial carbon dioxide tension.

5. ET carbon dioxide is affected by:
   - Atmospheric pressure 1% rise in pressure raises the $ETCO_2$ by 1%.
   - The nitrous oxide concentration. It absorbs light at 450 nm and the device will read it as if it were carbon dioxide.
   - The presence of water vapour, which condenses on the window of the sensor cells. This gives a false rise in carbon dioxide reading. Normally the gases are analysed dry so the reading of carbon dioxide is made as a % of carbon dioxide, oxygen and nitrogen or nitrous oxide with the water vapour absent.
   - Remember that the capnograph is measuring dry gases and the water vapour in the alveoli has been removed. Unless it has a built in correction all readings will be higher than alveoli gas concentrations.
   - Inhalation anaesthetic agents absorb light at 3300 nm but not enough to make a real difference.

6. Phase IV
   Rapid fall in carbon dioxide tension towards the baseline and fresh gas flow replaces alveoli gas at the sample port.

7. a. A rise in the base line occurs with:
   - Rebreathing.
   - Addition of carbon dioxide to the breathing system.
   - Incompetent expiratory valve.
   - Using a Bain system.

- Using a breathing system with inadequate fresh gas flow.
- Exhaustion of carbon dioxide absorption.

b. Sudden reduction in height of curve
  - Disconnection – check breathing system connections.
  - Fall in cardiac output – check pulse. Causes – emboli, bleeding, and cardiac arrest.

c. Gradually rising slope
  - Alveoli are emptying with different concentrations of carbon dioxide due to ventilation to perfusion inequalities.
  - Seen in COAD, bronchospasm, pulmonary oedema. May be seen with kyphoscoliois, which also gives a double hump as the lungs empty at different rates.
  - Obstruction to gas flow, tube partially blocked or kinked.

8. The sampling should be on the anaesthetic machine or ventilator side of the HME to eliminate water vapour from the tubing. It should be away from the fresh gas flow during expiration, which will dilute the expired carbon dioxide.

The sampling tubing should be small bore, < 2 mm diameter. Small bore tubing limits gas mixing, the introduction of foreign particles and limits the amount of gas taken out of the breathing system. The sampled gas should be returned to circuit.

The length of sample tubing should be < 2 m to give a fast response time and avoid distortion of the waveform.

Answers – Monitoring equipment 4

1. ▪ Variable orifice/constant pressure
     ● Rotameter
     ● Wright respirometer
   ▪ Fixed orifice/variable pressure
     ● Pneumotacograph
     ● Bourdon gauge
   ▪ Bubble flow meter
   ▪ Mass spectrometer.

2. Spirometers
   ▪ Dry – vitalograph
   ▪ Water seal – Benedict Roth Spirometer
   ▪ Dry gas meter
   ▪ Electronic volume meter.

3. Wright respirometer

   ▪ It is a variable orifice, constant pressure, flow meter.

4. It consists of a gas inlet and outlet. There is a cylinder containing a tube of many slanted foils. Gas is directed from the outside of the tube between the foils onto a central vane, which rotates. The centre of the vane is attached to a pointer to give the degree of rotation, which is proportional to the amount of gas flow.

5. Inaccuracies are due to the inertia of the vane.

   ▪ Over-reads at high flows
   ▪ Under-reads at low flows
   ▪ Most accurate at continuous flows proving calibration is reliable.

6. It measures flow in one direction only as the vane does not rotate in the reverse direction. It should be placed on the expiratory limb and as proximal to the patient as possible for the following reasons:

   ▪ The expiratory limb is working with lower pressures of gas flow.
   ▪ Any gas lost from the breathing system due to leaks or tubing expansion will not be counted in the measurement.
   ▪ It is more important to know what the patient has breathed out than what the ventilator delivered.

7. It is less accurate over time due to moisture and dirt particles, which cause sticking and increase resistance to rotation of the vanes.

8. The Wright's peak flow meter

9. The peak flow meter has a moveable vane. Air is blown into the box and against the vane. A slit in the perimeter of the base allows the air to escape. As more air is blown in so the more the vane rotates. The pointer moved by the vane stays fixed at the peak flow until reset.

10. A Pneumotacograph measures flow rate. Volume can be deduced as a function of flow and time.

11. A tube is made with a restriction in the lumen. Pressures are measured either side of the restriction. The flow rate is proportional to the pressure drop.

12. The gas flow is laminar and therefore calibration depends on the viscosity of the gas.

Notes on Wright's respirometer
- Variable orifice, constant pressure respirometer
- Measures gas volume
- Under reads at low flows <1 litre
- Affected by moisture which causes sticking
- One way system of air flow
- The slits create a circular flow to rotate the vane
- The vane makes 150 revolutions for 1 litre
- Placed proximally in the expiratory side of the breathing system
- Accuracy ± 5–10%
- Resistance 2 cm H_2O at 100 l/min

Notes on Pneumotacograph
- Measures flow rate and peak flow
- Affected by gas viscosity
- Fixed orifice, variable pressure
- Senses the change in pressure across a fixed resistance, gas flow is laminar
- Consists of a tube with a fixed resistance of one or a bundle of tubes
- Sensitive pressure transducers on either side of the resistance
- Bi-directional for measuring flow rate and tidal volume

Answers – Monitoring Equipment 5

1. **False** – It selectively measures the pulsatile component of light absorbed in the visible and near infrared spectra.

2. **False** – Two: 660 and 940 nm.

3. **False** – The saturation is taken as a mean over 5–10 beats.

4. **True** – Smokers' blood may contain high concentrations of carboxyhaemoglobin. This will tend to increase the measured oxygen saturation by about 50% of the percentage of carboxyhaemoglobin present.

5. **True** – Alkalosis shifts the oxyhaemoglobin dissociation curve to the left, increasing the affinity of haemoglobin for oxygen.

6. **False** – Because the apparatus relies on pulsatile light absorption, a low pulse pressure will render it less accurate.

7. **False** – Bilirubin does not affect the accuracy as its absorption peaks are at 460, 560 and 600 nm.

8. **False** – Due to the shape of the oxyhaemoglobin dissociation curve, the saturation starts to drop rapidly at 90% with the onset of hypoxia. Therefore the alarm should be set at 94% to detect the first signs of a reduction in saturation before it becomes fatal. Not 90% as set on this device, unless the patient has a degree of reduced oxygenation.

9. **True** – Especially in infants.

10. **False** – Arterial haemoglobin saturation will be normal in cyanide poisoning. Mixed venous saturation will be high due to reduced oxygen utilisation in the tissues.

MEASURING EQUIPMENT

7

Questions

1. What is the name of this apparatus and why is it so named? List at least two features that increase the accuracy of the reading.

2. What is illustrated at **B**?

3. Which formula describes the flow at **B**?

4. What is illustrated at **C**?

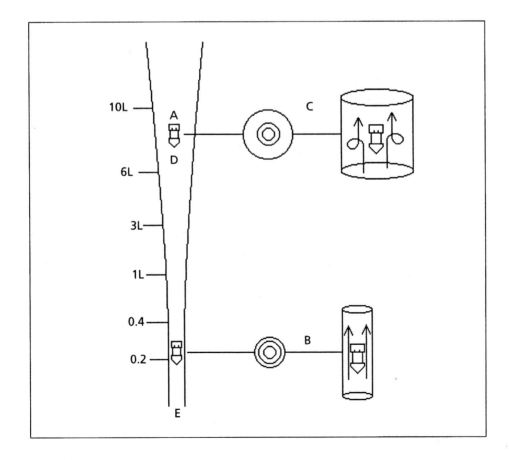

5. Which formulae describes the flow at **C**?

6. What describes the pressure difference between **A** and **D**?

7. What controls the flow at **E**?

8. When gas is flowing what is the pressure at **E**?

9. When could a rotameter be used accurately for two different gases?

10. What safety features are present on a modern Boyle's machine to prevent giving a hypoxia mixture?

Measuring equipment 2 *(Answers on page 225)*

Humidity

Questions

1. How is humidity defined?

2. Why should the humidity in theatre be between 50 and 70% at temperatures above 20°C?

3. How much does the absolute humidity increase by between room temperature of 20°C and intra-alveolar (body) temperature of 37°C?

4. How can relative humidity be measured?

5. Explain the principle underlying the way each works.

6. What is the dew point?

7. What changes occur in the body if inspired air is not humidified?

Measuring Equipment 3   *(Answers on page 229)*

Temperature

Questions – Part I

1. What is the normal body temperature?

2. Why is body temperature maintained at this level?

3. What is the device pictured opposite?

4. What is the scale and how is it graduated?

5. What are the advantages of using this device?

6. What are the disadvantages?

7. Where can body temperature be measured

8. What is core temperature?

9. Where can core temperature be measured?

10. What other fluid can be used in a thermometer?

11. What is the SI unit for temperature and how is it defined?

12. What is the triple point of water?

Questions – Part II

1. Name the different electrical principles for measuring clinical temperature.

2. What other means are available for measuring temperature?

3. What is the relationship between temperature and the electrical change for each of the electrical devices?

4. What are the advantages and disadvantages of each electrical method?

5. Where can body temperature be most accurately measured?

6. How is heat lost from the body?

7. As a percentage, which method of heat loss accounts for the greatest heat loss during anaesthesia?

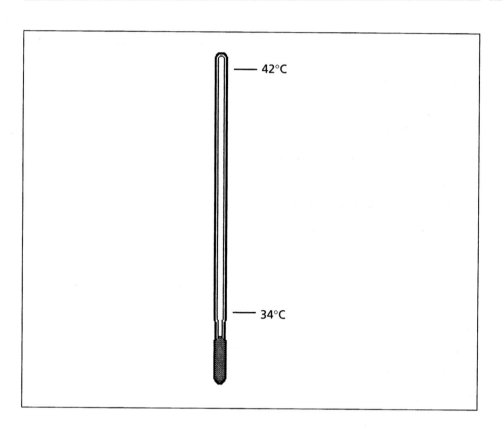

Measuring Equipment 4 *(Answers on page 233)*

Spirometer loop

Questions

1. What do loops 1 and 3 represent in the top figures?

2. Label the lines relating to inspiration and expiration?

3. What is compliance?

4. What is the difference between static and dynamic compliance?

5. What is the work of breathing?

6. What does loop 2 represent?

7. The bottom figures show a flow/volume loop taken with the patient breathing from a maximum expiration to a maximum inspiration. Label inspiration and expiration; the residual volume and the vital capacity; the peak inspiratory and peak expiratory flow rates. Draw the change in the curve with obstruction to inspiration and obstruction to expiration.

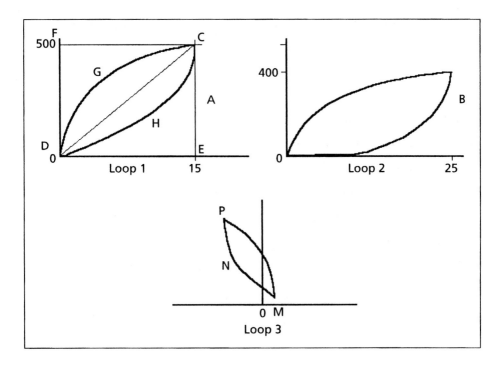

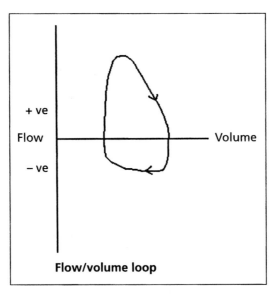

Flow/volume loop

8. **E, F, G** are three flow/volume loops. Indicate which is compatible with normal, emphysema and ankylosing spondylitis. Label the direction the trace moves and the expiratory and inspiratory phases.

9. What happens to the loop if there is a blockage of the tracheal tube with secretions?

10. What factors lead to a reduction in the functional residual capacity?

11. What are the bedside tests of pulmonary function?

12. What can be diagnosed from loops **H, I, J** and **K**?

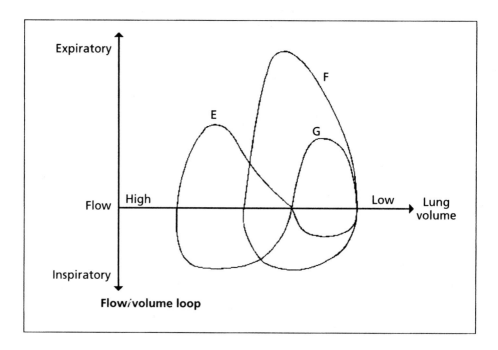

Flow/volume loop

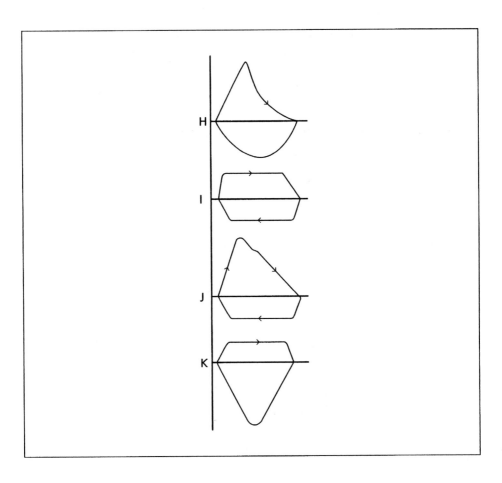

Measuring Equipment 5 *(Answers on page 235)*

Peripheral nerve stimulator

Questions

1. What range of voltage and current does a nerve stimulator give for transcutaneous testing of neuromuscular blockade? What might skin resistance be dry and wet?

2. How would you use this device to stimulate the ulnar nerve at the wrist? What are the landmarks and what response (which muscles contract) would be seen in the unparalysed patient?

3. How should the electrodes be placed on the patient?

4. Which other nerve/muscle groups can be used?

5. What is a supra maximal stimulus?

6. What is the muscle response to a nerve stimulator in a partial depolarising block?

7. What are the two phenomena shown in the figure opposite and what do the responses represent?

8. What percentage of receptors must be occupied by a competitive blocker before depression of the twitch?

9. What is a post-tetanic count?

10. When is it used?

11. What does a train of four mean and when can reversal drugs be given? What might be more useful than a train of four and why?

12. What would be the characteristics of the ideal nerve stimulator?

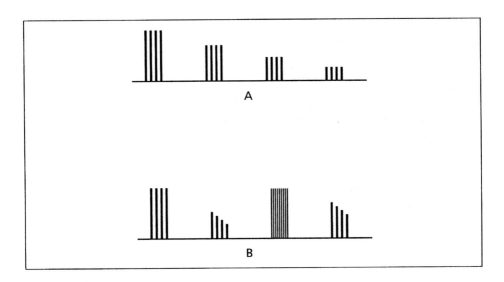

Measuring Equipment 6 *(Answers on page 237)*

Direct Blood pressure reading

Questions
1. How is the system illustrated opposite calibrated?

2. What types of transducer are available for use at **A**?

3. What are the principles of the Wheatstone bridge?

4. What are the problems with using a transducer for measuring pressure?

5. Draw the waveforms for a normal arterial trace, resonance and damping.

6. What is damping and how does it occur?

7. Diagram C shows four types of damping. What are they?

8. What is resonance and how does it occur?

9. What should be the characteristics of the tubing at **B**?

10. What is the fluid of choice for the intra-arterial flush at **C**?

11. What pressure is used in the flush bag at **D**?

12. What is the effect of air in the line?

13. What will happen if a 16 g venflon is used for the arterial cannula at **E**?

14. How can the zero affect the reading?

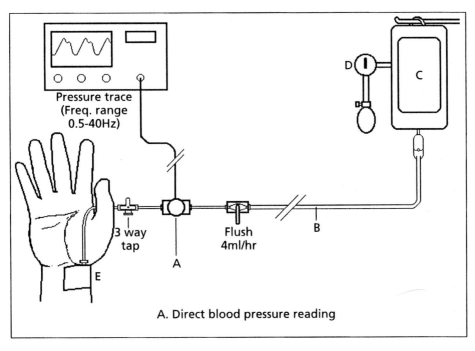

A. Direct blood pressure reading

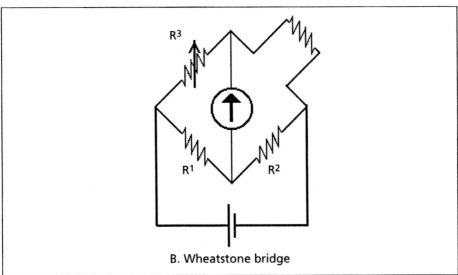

B. Wheatstone bridge

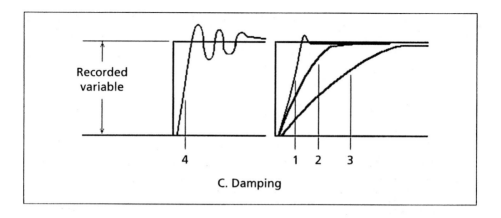

C. Damping

Answers
Measuring Equipment

Answers – Measuring Equipment 1

1. This is a rotameter to distinguish it from other flowmeters. The bobbin is fluted and rotates. The tube must be vertical. The inside is coated with a conductive material – a film of gold. This is connected to earth to prevent the accumulation of static electricity. If the bobbin sticks due to dirt or static it will not rotate. The reading is taken from the flat top of the bobbin as compared with the waist of a ball bobbin.

2. Laminar flow through a tube.

3. Flow is proportional to radius^4 × pressure difference / length × viscosity.

4. Turbulent flow through an orifice.

5. Flow^2 is proportional to pressure difference × radius^4/density.

6. The weight of the rotameter. The pressure across the bobbin remains constant because the weight is constant. The annular orifice increases with higher gas flows.

7. A needle valve.

8. The reduced pressure from the reducing valve or the pressure of the central supply coming from the wall pipes (400 kPa).

9. At low flow the viscosities would have to be similar, at high flow the density would have to be similar.

10. ■ Cylinders are pin-indexed and colour-coded.
    ■ The self-closing sockets on the wall have specific probes for specific gases and the tubing is colour-coded.
    ■ There is a link between the oxygen and the nitrous oxide rotameters to prevent less than 25% oxygen being given.
    ■ Oxygen failure warning device.

Notes on the rotameter

This is a constant pressure, variable orifice, rotating bobbin, flow meter.

The tube varies in diameter with the taper wider at the top. Some have a double taper.

Each tube is calibrated at: 1 atmosphere of pressure, room temperature, for a specific gas.

If the atmospheric pressure increases, the flow meter will over-read.

Gas with an increased viscosity will over-read at low flows.

Gas of increased density will over-read at high flows.

Ambient temperature changes make little difference to the reading.

A hypoxic mixture can be delivered if there is a:

- Leak at the top of the oxygen tube
- Oxygen flow meter upstream of other gases such as nitrous oxide.

Answers – Measuring Equipment 2

1. Humidity is defined in two ways

   ▪ Absolute humidity is the mass of water vapour present in a given volume of gas, at a defined temperature. It is expressed as g/m³ or g/l.
   ▪ Relative humidity is the ratio of the mass of water vapour present in a gas to the mass required to saturate that volume of gas at the same temperature.

2. If humidity is too low, static charge can build up leading to sparks.

   If the humidity is too high, it makes working conditions uncomfortable.

   The temperature is kept high to minimise heat loss from the patient. Humidity is related to temperature NOT pressure.

3. From 17 to 44 g/l or 27 g/l (see graph below).

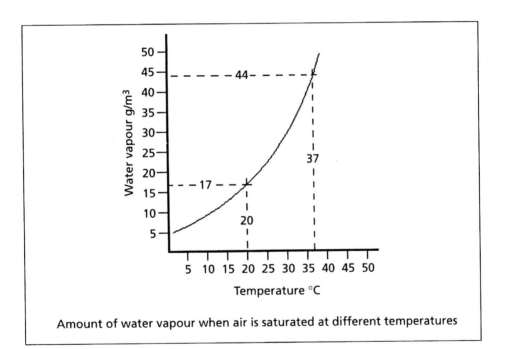

Amount of water vapour when air is saturated at different temperatures

4. *a.* Relative humidity can be measured using a:
  - Hair hygrometer (below)
  - Wet and dry bulb hygrometer (opposite – top)
  - Renault's hygrometer (opposite – bottom)

  b. Absolute humidity can be measured using a:
  - Humidity transducer
  - Mass spectrometer.

5. ■ The Hair hygrometer. A hair increases in length as humidity increases. Simple and accurate between about 15 and 85% humidity.
  ■ Wet and dry hygrometer. Two mercury thermometers side by side. One bulb measures room temperature and a wick soaked in water surrounds the other bulb. This bulb is cooled by the evaporation of the water. The lower the humidity the more evaporation occurs causing the temperature to fall. The relative humidity is determined by entering the two temperatures onto predetermined tables.
  ■ Regnault's hygrometer. A tube with a silver outer lining is filled with ether and a thermometer. Pumping air through the ether, which evaporates, cools the air surrounding the silver lining. When the ether cools to the temperature at which the surrounding air is totally saturated, water condenses on the silver tube. This is the Dewpoint. Tables are used to calculate the humidity at the room temperature, knowing the dew point temperature at which the air is fully saturated with water vapour.

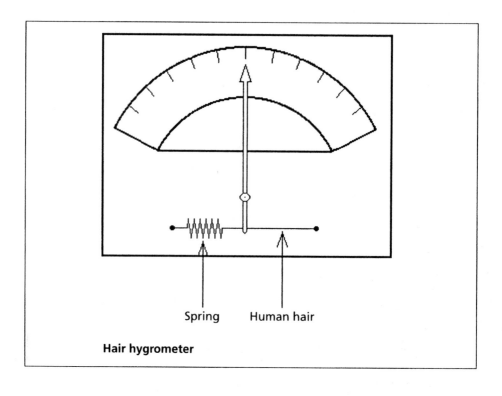

Spring   Human hair

Hair hygrometer

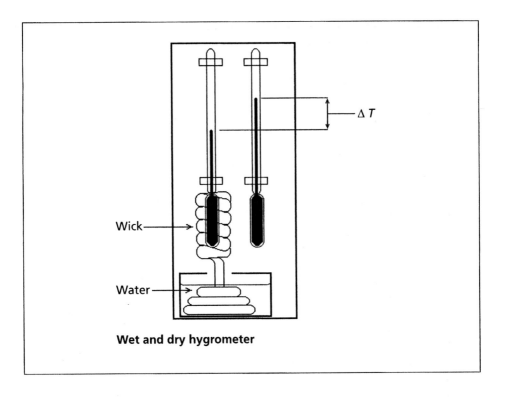

Wet and dry hygrometer

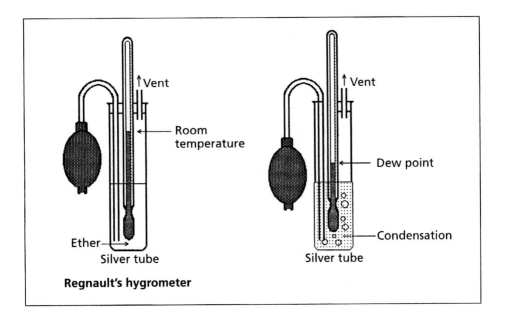

Regnault's hygrometer

- The humidity transducer measures the change in resistance or capacitance when silica gel absorbs water. This gives a very sensitive device.
- The mass spectrometer. Measurement is based on the absorption of ultraviolet light by water vapour.

6. The dew point is the temperature at which the air is fully saturated with water vapour and condensation occurs.

7. Inspired dry air leads to:

- Desquamation of cells and squamous metaplasia.
- Loss of cilia function and then loss of cilia.
- Increased viscosity of sputum and mucus plugging of airways.
- Reduced compliance and increased airway resistance.
- Loss of surfactant.
- Atelectasis and increased shunt.
- Reduced FRC.
- Hypothermia.

Answers – Measuring Equipment 3

Part I

1. 37°C.

2. To optimise the function of enzyme pathways.

3. Mercury clinical thermometer.

4. 34–42°C. Graduated by placing in two known temperatures and drawing a linear scale between the two fixed points.

5. Advantages:
   a. Reliable. Mercury thermometer relies on the low thermal conductivity of mercury. This means that the increase in volume of mercury with increase in temperature is linear over the range of body temperature. Mercury solidifies at −39°C and boils at + 200°C.
   b. Accurate. The mercury is contained in a very thin column so that the readings are spread out along a length of the tube. This thin column is kept short by limiting the range of readings. A constriction at the bottom of the column fixes the expanded column for reading, until the mercury is shaken down past the constriction. A silver backing aids reading and a curved lens-like front magnifies the reading.
   c. Cheap for general ward use.

6. Disadvantages:
   a. Slow response time. It may take 2–3 minutes to equilibrate.
   b. It cannot be used in all orifices and even in the mouth may be inaccurate if the patient cannot breathe through their nose and breathes cold air over the mercury.
   c. It can break, with the problems of spilling glass and mercury.

7. Temperature can be measured in the nose, external auditory meatus, mouth, oesophagus, pulmonary artery flotation catheter from the right atrium to the pulmonary artery and the rectum.

8. Core temperature is central body temperature or the temperature of blood at the hypothalamus. It is the temperature of the blood in the vital organs: heart, lung and the brain.

9. Core temperature can be approximated to by measurements in the:
   - Lower third of the oesophagus
   - Nasopharynx
   - External auditory meatus
   - Pulmonary artery flotation catheter in the right side of the heart
   - Urinary bladder with a probe on a catheter.

10. Alcohol. It is cheap and more suitable for very low temperatures but not high temperatures as it boils at 78°C.

11. SI unit – degrees Kelvin: 1 Kelvin is 1/273 of the thermodynamic temperature of the triple point of water.

12. Triple point of water is when ice, water and water vapour are in equilibrium or 0°Celsius, 273°Kelvin.

Part II

1. Electrical methods:

- Thermistor – resistance change
- Thermocouple – potential difference change
- Platinum – resistance change.

2. Other methods:

- Crystal colour change
- Coiled tube expansion – elliptical coil of metal (similar to an anaeroid barometer) expands as heat is applied in side or outside.
- Bimetallic strip in dial thermometer.

3. Graphs
  a. Thermistor metal oxide, which acts as a semiconductor. Resistance of oxide **falls** exponentially with increases in temperature.
  b. Thermocouple. When the join between two different metals is heated a potential difference is created which has a linear relationship to the degree of heating (Seebeck effect). The two metals are copper and an alloy of copper with nickel. One electrode is kept at a constant temperature as a reference electrode. The other is used as the temperature probe.
  c. Platinum resistance change. The electrical resistance of a metal – platinum – increases linearly with increases in temperature.

4. *a.* Thermistor. Advantages – Cheap to produce, large resistance changes. Disadvantage – Problem with calibration.
  b. Thermocouple. Advantage – Fast response time 0.1 to 10 seconds, made in the form of a needle probe.
  c. Platinum resistance change. Disadvantage – Not very sensitive as amount of change in resistance is not great for each degree of temperature change.

5. Tympanic membrane is unaffected by other factors.

Breathing may cool nasal air and to a lesser extent oesophageal temperature may be distorted by the cooler air in the trachea.

Rectal temperature may be affected by the presence of faeces.

6. Heat is lost by:

- Conduction. Heat is transferred from a high temperature object to a low temperature object. The skin warms the air over it.
- Convection. Warm air is less dense so rises away from the skin to be replaced by cooler air.
- Radiation. Does not require matter. This way heat is lost from all bodies and travels through space.

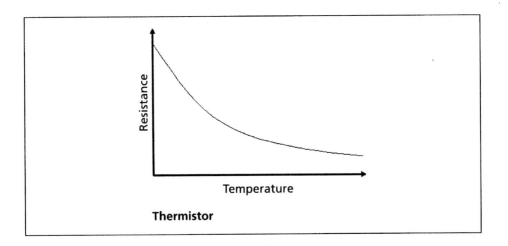

Thermistor

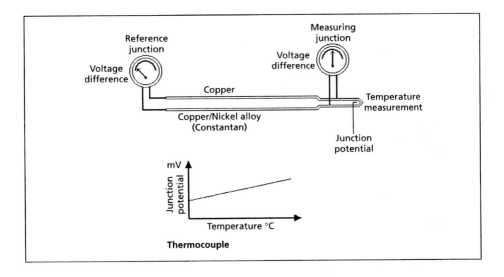

Thermocouple

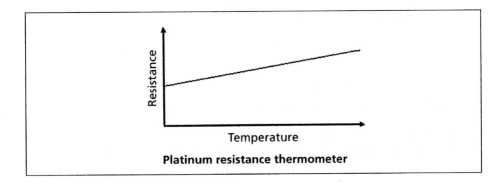

Platinum resistance thermometer

■ Evaporation. Water is converted to vapour using up a lot of calories. The latent heat of vaporisation.

7. Radiation 40%, Convection 30%, Evaporation 30%.

Answers – Measuring Equipment 4

1. These are pressure–volume loops. Loop 1 is a patient ventilated by IPPV and 3 is a spontaneously breathing patient.

2. Inspiratory flow is along OHC and MNP.

3. Compliance = volume/unit pressure.

   Total compliance = Tidal volume 500 ml/5 cm H_2O = 100 ml/cm H_2O.

4. Static compliance measures the pressure and volume at the beginning and again at the end of inspiration and subtracts the one from the other. Dynamic compliance takes into account the curve of the loop and integrates the area between the loop and the straight line CD.

5. Work = Force × distance.

   As Pressure = Force/area, then F = PA.

   Volume = Distance × Area, so Distance = Volume/Area.

   So combining the equations Work = PA (Force) × V/A (Distance), so Work = P × V.

   The work of inspiration is the pressure change × the volume moved

   1 kPa x 0.5 m³ = 0.5 Joules.

6. Curve of obstruction. A more rectangular shaped curve due to a higher pressure to deliver air into the lung. Due to a partially obstructed tube, bronchospasm, pulmonary oedema.

7.

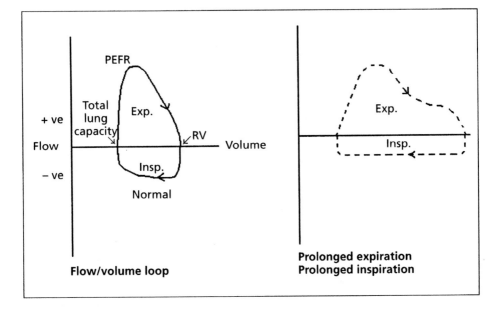

Flow/volume loop

Prolonged expiration
Prolonged inspiration

8. Flow/volume loop:

Loop **E** is emphysema.

Loop **F** is normal.

Loop **G** is ankylosing spondylitis.

9. The expiratory line (where **F** is marked) will be a serrated edge as air flows past the secretions.

10. Functional residual capacity decreases with:
   a. anaesthesia
   b. from sitting to supine position

FRC increases with age.

11. Hold inspiration for > 30 seconds, blow out a flame at 15 cm with open mouth. Vitalograph used to give spirometer values depending on how the patient breathes.
   a. Tidal volume, inspiratory and expiratory reserve volumes, vital capacity.
   b. Forced expiratory volume and forced expiratory volume in 1 second.

From Wright's peak flow meter:
   a. Peak expiratory flow rate.

From electronic spirometer
   a. Volume pressure loops
   b. Flow volume loops.

Respiratory muscle strength. Pressure generated by inspiration against a closed glottis.

12.
   H. Small airway obstruction.
   I. Fixed obstruction e.g. tracheal stenosis
   J. Variable extrathoracic obstruction e.g. cord palsy
   K. Variable intrathoracic obstruction e.g. tracheomalacia.

Answers – Measuring Equipment 5

1. Battery power 3 to 9 volts. Skin resistance dry 1000 ohms, wet 100 ohms. I = V/R. Current with dry skin 1 to 10 milliamps, wet skin 100 milliamps.

2. In practice, if the nerve stimulator has no output control, it can only be used on the unconscious patient, as currents over 1 milliamp are painful. On a conscious patient only use a stimulator with a current regulator. Explain to the patient that there will be paraesthesia and a muscle twitch. Obtain their consent.

   The ulnar nerve lies between palmaris longus and flexor carpi ulnaris. Or to the medial side of the mid-point of the wrist on the ventral surface, proximal to the wrist skin crease.

   Stimulation of the nerve causes the hypothenar muscles to contract with strong flexion of the little finger due to contraction of the flexor digitorum brevis, the lumbrical and interossei; less flexion of the ring finger due to interossei and lumbrical contraction. Much less flexion of the middle and index fingers due to the interossei muscles only innervated by the ulnar nerve to these two fingers. The thumb adducts due to contraction of adductor pollucis brevis, one of the thenar muscles.

3. Apply a small amount of electrolyte containing gel to reduce the skin resistance, electrode either small ECG type or ball covered with conducting gel. Negative pole placed distally over the nerve and the positive pole on the skin 2 cm proximally or away from nerve.

   Check stimulus strength if patient awake before switching on. Select mode: single twitch, 50 Hz, TOF, double burst or tetanus.

   Measure response by observation of contraction, palpate contraction, or transducer for pressure.

4. Facial nerve as it leaves the styloid foramen by the mastoid bone or as it passes through the parotid gland. Common peroneal or lateral popliteal nerve at the head of the fibula. Posterior tibial nerve behind the medial malleolus.

5. A supra maximal stimulus is used to stimulate a peripheral nerve through the skin. The current is sufficiently high to ensure that all the motor nerves are depolarised. A nerve stimulator is powered by a 3 to 9 volt battery. The resistance of the skin is normally 100–1000 ohms. So the current will be I = V/R or I = 6 volts/100–1000 ohms = 6–60 milliamps. If an electrode gel is used to reduced skin resistance, the current will always be above 50 milliamps. The duration is usually 0.2–1.0 millisecond.

6. Reduced magnitude of twitch response to a tenanus or ToF stimulus.

7. *a.* Non-depolarising block.
   b. Fade and post-tetanic potentiation.

8. 75%.

9. A tetanus will increase the amount of acetyl choline available and so enhance the next response. The post-tetanic count is the number of twitches that are visible following a tetanic burst.
10. To monitor profound neuromuscular blockade.
11. A train of four equal twitches are four supramaximal stimuli at 2 Hz. Four twitches means complete recovery, three responses means only 25% recovery and reversal can be given with care. Two twitches 20%, and one twitch 10% recovery. This is not enough to reverse to good power. Double bursts of three stimuli at 50 Hz followed after 0.75 seconds by two or three more stimuli at 50 Hz. It is easier to compare the two responses.
12. Portable, battery-operated, rechargeable, leads that can be sterilised, optimum pulse duration 0.25 milliseconds, range of pulses: monophasic, rectangular, square wave, variable current output 20–50 milliamps.

Answers – Measuring Equipment 6

1. The system is calibrated by choosing:
   a. One low point – zero.
   b. One high point – 100 mmHg.

2. The transducers commonly in use are based on:
   a. Change in resistance of metal mounted as an arm of a Wheatstone bridge.
   b. Change of resistance of piezo-electric crystal.
   c. Change of capacitance of two metal diaphragms acting as a capacitor.

3. The Wheatstone bridge consists of four resistances arranged in a rectangle. A current is applied to the circuit and a very sensitive galvanometer detects any difference in the resistance between each pair of resistors.

   One resistor is used as the measuring part. The bridge is used in two ways. Either a variable resistance is adjusted to give no current flow in the circuit and that change in the variable resistance is the measure of change; or the change in the galvanometer is taken as the measure of change.

4. Damping and resonance.

5.

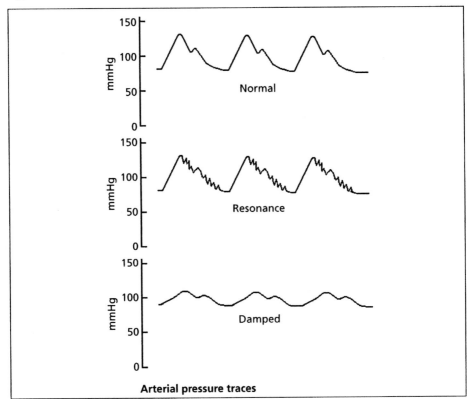

Arterial pressure traces

6. Damping is the tendency of a system to **resist** the **oscillation** caused by sudden change. The arterial pressure is continually changing and the movement of the pulse is transmitted to the column of fluid leading to the transducer. The pressure in the fluid column will tend to oscillate with a frequency, which is a harmonic of the pulse pressure.

   The natural frequency of the column. If this is less than 40 Hz its falls within the range of the blood pressure and a sine wave will be superimposed on the blood pressure wave.

7. Resonance
   1. Optimal. This is 0.6–0.7 or critical damping. It has minimal amplitude distortion and minimal pulse delay. It produces the fastest response without excessive oscillation.
   2. Critical. The system is said to be critically damped when D = 1. There is a rapid change in pressure with no over-shoot of the trace.
   3. Over-damped D >>1. There is an excessively delayed response.

   The wave form is flat, falsely low systolic and high diastolic, the mean is unchanged.

   Damping is due to: narrow tubing, long elastic tube, high density of fluid, compliant diaphragm and tubing, air bubbles in the fluid, which will absorb some of the pressure changes, clot formation.
   4. Under-damped D<<1. Marked over-shoot followed by oscillations. Leads to falsely high systolic and low diastolic readings, the mean is unchanged.

8. Resonance occurs when an oscillating system responds with maximum amplitude to an alternating external driving force.

   This occurs when the driving frequency coincides with the natural frequency. Then the system starts to oscillate and the magnitude of the wave form is magnified.

9. The system frequency is made higher by: large bore tubing, short length of tubing, stiff wall catheter, low density fluid, stiff diaphragm.

10. Dextrose is used as a non-electrical conducting fluid to avoid a current passing down the catheter into the heart.

11. The pressure is kept at 300 mmHg or 50% above systolic pressure to provide a flush to keep the line free of blood which may clot.

12. Air in the system will lead to damping.

13. If the calibre of the inter-arterial cannula is too large the system will be under-damped.

14. The zero must rise and fall when the patient is moved for accurate readings.

ANAESTHETIC HAZARDS

8

Notes on electricity and electrical safety

Explain static electricity.
Friction between two non-conducting bodies results in electron transfer from one to the other. The body, which gains electrons, becomes relatively negative and possesses potential energy. An electrical potential difference develops between the two bodies. If there are particles in the air, such as moisture they will reduce the build up of surface electrons.

Static is a source of sparks which can lead to theatre fires and explosions.

What is an atom?
An atom is composed of a central nucleus around which electrons revolve in an orbit. Electrons are of small mass and negatively charged. The nucleus is of large mass protons, positively charged and an equal mass of neutrons without charge. The mass of 1840 electrons equals the mass of 1 proton.

A normal atom contains equal numbers of protons and electrons.

The maximum number of electrons in a particular orbit can be calculated:

Number $= 2 \times n^2$ (n = number of orbit from nucleus).

The electrons in the outer orbit are *valent electrons.*

They determine the chemical properties of the atom.

If energy such as heat, light or electricity is applied to an electron it absorbs it and jumps from an orbit near to the nucleus to one further away.

What is a conductor?
In a conductor, the outer orbit electrons are loosely bound to the nucleus. They can readily move through the substance under the influence of an electrical potential. Such substances are metals, carbon and liquid including saline and body fluids.

What is an insulator?
The outer electrons are firmly bound to the nucleus. They are not normally able to move to create a potential difference. Such substances are glass, rubber and mica.

What is a semiconductor?

This is a substance that is halfway between a conductor and an insulator. The outer orbit of electrons is bound to the atoms less firmly than an insulator thereby giving the electron a little extra energy. It can escape from the atom to which it is bound and can conduct electricity, e.g. Thermistor. Heat is the source of energy; as the temperature rises more electrons escape.

A photodetector is a special type of semiconductor in the form of a resistor, a diode and a transistor.

When radiation falls on the detector, electrons absorb some of the energy of the radiation and are able to move through the materials more freely.

How is a magnetic field created?

A conductor with a current flowing through it can exert a force on another conductor carrying current. This property is known as magnetism.

It is due to the sum of the many minute currents formed by the motion of the electrons orbiting their nuclei, e.g. iron.

A magnetic field is the region throughout which a magnet or a current-carrying conductor exerts its effect. Changing the magnetic field induces a flow of electrons in a conductor to produce an electric current.

An electric current is a flow of electrons.

The rate of flow of electrical charge is measured in amperes. 1 ampere = a charge of 1 coulomb flowing for 1 second.

1 ampere represents a flow of 6.24×10^{18} electrons per second past a point.

A current can be produced by negative or positive charges.

Whenever an electric current flows in a wire an associated magnetic field exists around the wire.

Equally, whenever a wire carrying an electric current is placed in a magnetic field there is a force on the wire which tends to move the wire in a direction perpendicular to the electrical current and the magnetic field.

The interaction between an electric current and a magnetic field is the working principle behind devices such as a galvanometer and the cause of interference.

Describe the differences between DC and AC current.

There are two types of electrical current

- Direct current (DC)
- Alternating current (AC).

Direct current is a steady flow of electrons along a wire or through a component in one direction. Sources: Thermocouple. Battery – a chemical energy is converted into electrical energy through a chemical reaction.

Alternating current is the flow of electrons first in one direction and then in the other opposite direction along a wire.

AC can be represented as a sine wave, which has a wavelength. This is the distance between successive complete cycles.

Frequency is the number of waves per second (measured as Hertz or cycles per second).

In an electrical circuit, electrons flow from the negatively charged cathode to the positively charged anode BUT the current is said to flow from the anode to the cathode.

- *Coulomb*
- SI unit of charge
- The quantity of electrical charge which passes a point when a current of one ampere flows for one second.
- It is an amount of electricity equivalent to 6.24×10^{18} electrons.

Ohm ( )
- The unit of electrical resistance.
- The resistance which allows one ampere of current to flow under the influence of a potential of one volt.

Definitions to learn
Resistance R = potential V / current I

When electrical charge flows through a resistor, energy is dissipated and the resistor heats up.

Work
 Work done = applied force $\times$ distance moved.
 Force = electromotive force.
 Distance = amount of charge which is moved.

$E = VI_t$
 Or electrical power (rate of work) 1 Watt = VI.

Work is measured in Joules J

Power is measured in Watts W

The heating effect in electrical equipment with a fixed resistance increases in proportion to:

- Square of the supply current
- Square of the current drawn out.

Voltage
 1 volt is the potential difference, which produces a current of 1 ampere in a substance when the rate of energy dissipated is 1 Watt.

 Volt V = Power Watts / Current A
 Power W = Energy J/second.
 Current A = charge C/second.

The energy delivered by a fixed amount of charge reduces as the voltage decreases.

UK current is 240 volts, 50 Hz. US 110 V, 60 Hz

A capacitor is a body able to hold electrical charge.

Two conductive plates separated by a insulator.

Capacitance is the measure of the ability to store energy.

Capacitors are found in:
> Pressure transducers. Defibrillators where they store the charge. A capacitor can be created when an operating theatre light acts as one plate and the patient acts as another plate causing interference, e.g. defibrillators.

What is a capacitor and how can it cause ECG interference?
A capacitor is two plates, which are not connected but store energy from an AC current. High frequency AC current passes easier than low frequency. DC current does not pass at all. Capacitors are used to model the storage of drugs as they might be distributed in the body by using theoretical circuits, in transducers and in defibrillators. A unit of capacitance is a FARAD: 1 farad is the capacitance when 1 coulomb is held by the plates with 1 volt difference between the plates.

The current flow through a capacitor is proportional to the rate of change of the voltage not the voltage itself. Any electrical device, powered by AC current can act as one plate of a capacitor and a patient acts as the other plate. This will cause a current with AC frequency to flow in the leads of an ECG.

What is an inductor and inductance?
An inductor is a coil of wire. Inductance is the resistance induced in a coil due to electo magnetic forces produced when a current flows through a wire or coil. It induces a magnetic field around the wire. This magnetic field is directly proportional to the current.

The magnetic field induces an EMF (potential difference or voltage) which is opposite in direction to the flow of current.

Inductance introduces a kind of inertia into the circuit.

Every time the current is switched off or on, the magnetic field lags behind and a back EMF is created in a direction opposite to the original current. This creates a frequency dependent resistance called *reactance in the conductor.*

Low frequency AC current passes more easily than high frequency (the opposite to a capacitor).

The importance of inductance
- Inductors are used in transducers.
- Inductance coupling. Many electrical devices have coils of wire with strong magnetic fields around them, e.g. transformers.
- This magnetic field will cause interference in adjacent apparatus. And in systems that are detecting small biological signals such as ECG monitors.

What is electrical interference?

Interference is the distortion of a biological signal. Caused by:

- Capacitance effects.
- Inductance effects.

Reduced by screening:

- The monitor leads are enclosed in a sheath of woven material, which is earthed. Interference currents are induced in the metal screen and not in the monitoring leads.
- The screening layer may be covered by a second layer of insulation.

What is resistance?

Resistance is a restriction to the movement of electrons in a DC circuit. Unit Ohms. When a DC current of 1 ampere produces a p.d. of 1 volt there is a resistance of 1 ohm.

Resistance increases when a wire is stretched to be long and thin. Heat increases the resistance in metals but reduces it in semiconductors.

Uses:

- Transducers
- Resistance in a Wheatstone bridge. The diaphragm in a pressure transducer moves, which alters the resistance in a wire (strain gauge).

The Wheatstone bridge has four resistances in balance. One is the sensing resistance. A change in current is a measure of the change in resistance. A variable resistance can be used to balance the system and the change in this variable resistance becomes the measure of change.

What is impedance?

Impedance is a measure of the hindrance to AC current flow through a capacitor. It is similar to resistance. The word resistance is applied to DC currents, whereas impedance is applied to AC currents. Impedance is made up of:

- Simple resistance
- A component that is inversely proportional to the frequency of AC current (the reactance).

It is not constant.

- DC current switches on, the current flow falls to zero, the p.d.(voltage) across the capacitor rises.
- AC current is constantly switched on and off. There is no steady state. The current flows through the capacitor but 90° after the voltage change. The current flow is proportional to the rate of voltage change.
- The reactance is inversely proportional to the frequency of the AC current.
- The resistance and the reactance combined give the opposite to current flow called the impedance.

Tissue impedance can be used to measure the change in composition in the tissue as impedance depends on the constituents of the tissue. Impedance is used for measuring:

- Carbon monoxide
- Spirometery
- Gastric emptying
- Limb plethysmography.

Skin impedance affects:

- The conduction of biological signals (ECG) through the skin to the electrode
- Attenuation of the signal.

Attenuation is reduced by reducing skin impedance by good electrical contact using electrolyte conductive gel and good adhesion.

What is the function of an electrical filter?
- Filters limit a signal to a small frequency range.
- Capacitive/resistive circuits filter out low frequencies. At high frequencies the impedance is low.
- Inductive circuits filter out high frequencies
- An inductive/capacitance circuit (band pass filters) only passes frequencies near the resonance frequency.

What is a transformer?
A transformer is made of two coils around a common iron core. It changes one voltage to another depending on the number of windings in each coil.

What are the characteristics of UK mains electricity?
It is supplied from generating stations at high voltage, 11 kV to make transfer of large amount of electricity easier. Reduced to 240 volts by local transformers, frequency 50 Hz.

Colour coding at socket:
Live – Brown, Neutral – Blue, Earth – Yellow/green.

What are the dangers of mains current?
- Electrocution
  Cardiac muscle is particularly sensitive to 50 Hz, which will cause VF.
- Macro shock through skin.
  1mA tingling, Over 1 mA pain, 15 mA and 50 Hz cases tonic contraction of striated muscle and person can not let go of the AC source. Death due to paralysis of respiratory muscles. 50 mA respiratory arrest, 100 mA VF. A current of 5 amp causes tonic contraction of the myocardial muscle as in defibrillation.
- Micro shock
  Direct myocardial contact of 150 micro amp. As the current density increases the voltage to give a shock falls, so current from a battery of 12 volts can give a micro shock.

Caused by leakage currents. That is a current not flowing in the designed direction.

Equipment intended for use with the heart must be of BS 5724 type CF or IEC 601-2-4 standard. It should have:

- Maximum leakage current of < 50 microamp, even with a single fault.
- Floating circuit.
- Low ionic liquid in the system (5% dextrose rather than 0.9% saline) in connections to the patient.

Shock is reduced by increasing skin impedance, which is normally 10–100 ohms.

Wet skin has low impedance.

Insulated footwear and antistatic floors.

VF is more likely if electrical shock occurs.

With early T wave, at 50 Hz, with myocardial disease or arrhythmias.

- Burns at point of high current density.
- Ignition of flammable materials due to heating effect of high current density.

How is electrical safety maintained in the operating theatre?
- Regularly check and service equipment by trained personnel.
- Inspect for obvious damage.
- Only use devices of the correct standard.

What are the classes of safety for electrical devices?
1. Class I earthed metal casing.
   Accidental contact between the live wire and the casing causes a large current to flow to earth – a fuse melts.
   A fuse is a thin wire offering a resistance, which melts when a current flows. It does not melt immediately so a current has passed and may cause damage.
2. Class II equipment
   Double insulation of all wires within the equipment. No earth required.
3. Class III internally powered either by battery or a transformer to reduce current to <24 volts.

- An isolated circuit (floating circuit) is an earth-free circuit.
- Uses diathermy, ECG monitors.
- The patient is connected to earth only through a transformer.

Leakage currents are due to drops in potential along a conductor.

Leakage current is detected and current flow stopped by a current-operated **Earth Leakage Circuit Breaker** (ELCB).

Standards for leakage currents are:

- Class BF surface contact, leak <100 microamp.
- Class CF maximum leak 10 microamp.

Minimise shock by:

- Keeping wires as short as possible.
- Avoiding trolleys passing over wires on floor.
- Carrying with dry hands.
- Avoiding extension boxes.
- No plugs on the floor.

Residual current circuit breaker (RCCB)

Allows current to flow while the current in the neutral wire is the same as in the live wire, i.e. no current flowing to earth by another route.

When there is a difference in the current between live and neutral of > 30 milliamp the RCCB opens and the current flow is switched off until reset.

Self-test: Diathermy
(Answers on page 253)

Questions: Part I

1. What are the component parts of a device to produce a diathermy current?

2. What is the principle of working of diathermy?

3. What is important about the pad?

4. There are three types of diathermy current. What are they and how do they differ? Draw the waveform of each.

5. What is the frequency of the current and why?

6. The diathermy can be used with and without a pad. What are these two modes of operation?

7. Name the parts of the **diagram** marked.

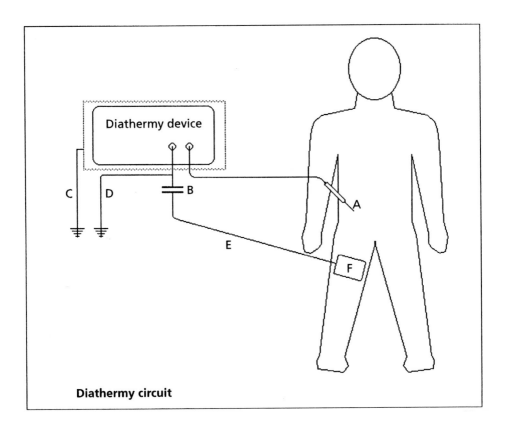

Diathermy circuit

8. What are the potential problems or hazards to the patient of using a diathermy?

9. Why does a diathermy not normally induce cardiac dysrhythmia, ventricular fibrillation or cardiac arrest?

10. What should be done before increasing the diathermy output?

11. When might a diathermy be used with a pacemaker device?

12. What is the code on a pacemaker and what does it mean?

Questions – Part II

1. State Ohm's Law.

2. The amount of heat produced in a circuit depends on the current and the resistance in the part where the heat is produced. What is the relationship between these parameters?

3. What are the parameters for mains electrical supply?

4. How is electrical apparatus used in operating theatres made electrically safe?

Self-test: Defibrillator   *(Answers on page 257)*

Questions

1. What are the potential electrical risks to the patient shown below?

2. What is the least amount of current that can do harm?

3. What is the effect of different currents passed into the body?

4. What do the International (IEC 601-1 1988) electrical symbols shown on page 250 mean?

5. What are the missing names or values in the electrical diagram of the defibrillator, shown on page 251?

6. What is the charge stored in the capacitor?

7. What is the function of the inductor?

8. What is a coulomb?

9. Why is the output from the defibrillator less than the peak charge?

10. What is the output from the defibrillator when switched on?

11. What is the waveform of the current and its duration?

12. What is the effect of this current on the heart?

13. When should the current be applied for the best effect?

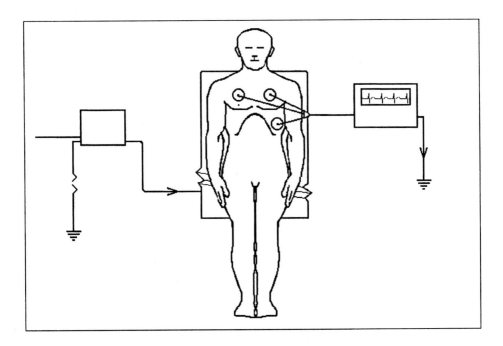

14. Why is a DC current used?

15. How should the paddles be used for defibrillation?

16. What is the size of the paddles?

17. What are the problems with defibrillation?

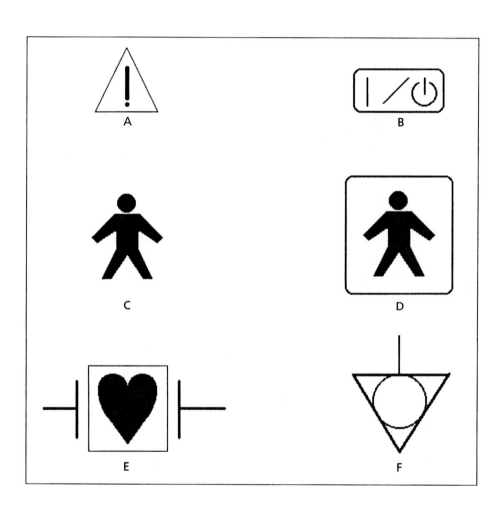

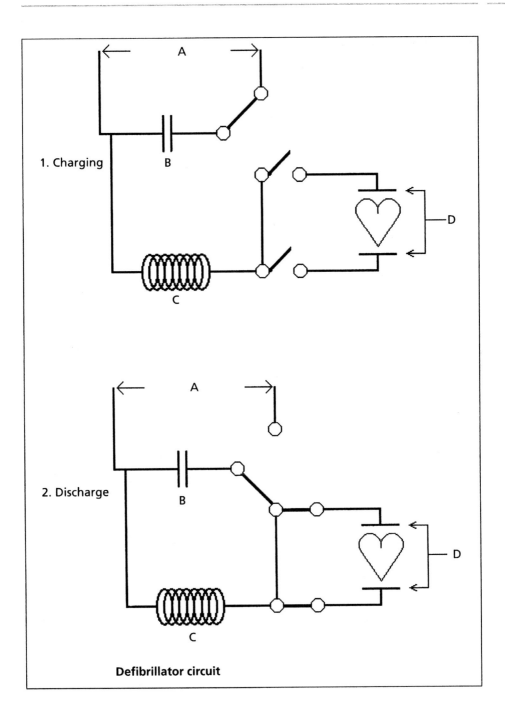

1. Charging

2. Discharge

Defibrillator circuit

Answers
Anaesthetic Hazards

Answers – Self-test: Diathermy

Part I

1. Features of a diathermy:
   - Device producing a controlled electrical output
   - Wire to patient
   - Pad and return wire.

2. Principle of operation

   When an electric current meets a high resistance there is a heating effect. The high resistance is where the needlepoint makes contact with the tissue. There is a high current density caused by the small area of contact between the needlepoint and tissue. The current returns out of the body through the large area pad with a low current density, so little heating effect.

3. Pad – large surface area, attached to skin with low electrical resistance, avoid hairy irregular surfaces. Size of indifferent electrode should fit patient, i.e. largest possible electrode for the patient but do not use an adult pad on a child or visa versa. Current density is the current flow per unit area. The same amount of current flows. Where the density is high heating occurs.

4. Cutting, coagulation and pulsed for coagulation.

A Cutting. A current that is alternating or a sine wave (sinusoidal wave). It is continuously oscillating and high frequency.

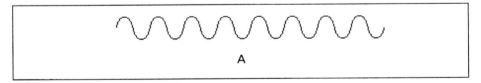

A

B Coagulation. A current that is damped.

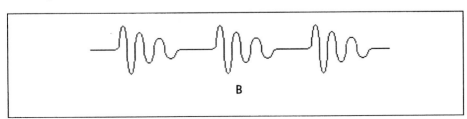

B

C Coagulation. A pulsed sine wave of 0.6 MHz in bursts of 20 seconds every 30 seconds.

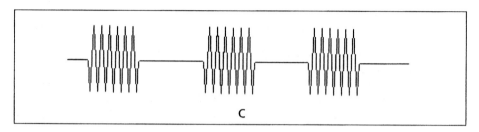

5. High frequency 5 kHz to 1.5 MHz. Alternating current to reduce stimulation and hence contraction of muscle.

6. Mono- and bipolar diathermy

Monopolar uses two electrodes remote from each other. The indifferent electrode is the pad plate, which should have a large surface area. The active electrode is a needlepoint to produce a high current density.

A bipolar diathermy uses two electrodes, which are the arms of the forceps.

The current flows between the tips of the arms. The bipolar diathermy is the safer to use with a pacemaker.

7. *A.* Active electrode.
  B. Isolating low impedance capacitance.
  C. Represents an isolated or floating patient circuit where the power supply is only connected to the patient circuit through an inductance coil.
  D. Earth.
  E. Indifferent electrode.
  F. Large area pad.

8. *a.* Electrocution
  b. Burns if
  ▪ Pad not applied to a large area of skin.
  ▪ Pad is not attached or badly attached the return current will flow through any point that the patient touches which will conduct electricity to earth: the metal of the table, metal touching the table or saline/blood-soaked drapes.
  ▪ Active electrode is accidentally switched on while touching any skin part. Keep the forceps in an insulated sheath.
  c. Interfere with:
  ▪ ECG signal on monitor
  ▪ Pulse oximeter
  ▪ Pacemaker function.

d. Fires and explosions have occurred due to:
- Flammable cleaning solutions
- Gas in bowel.

9. The diathermy current is a high frequency in the range of 1 Mhz. Living nerve and muscle tissue is sensitive to frequencies around 50 Hz. Fibrillation is most likely to occur with an AC current of about 50 Hz. Cardiac muscle stand still is induced by a DC current of a large potential across the heart as supplied in a defibrillator. With a diathermy, the exit from the body is controlled and the current passes in and out of the body between two electrodes.

The diathermy applied directly to muscle will cause contraction.

10. The active electrode should be cleaned. The contact of the indifferent electrode pad should be checked. The patient should be checked that there is no point of contact for a leakage current.

11. If the current field passes through the line of the pacemaker it may affect the function of a demand pacemaker. The pacemaker wire can act as an aerial and is affected by the electromagnetic field produced by the diathermy. The pacemaker may then interpret the diathermy current as a QRS complex. A demand pacemaker will stop functioning, particularly if the diathermy field is within 15 cm of the pacemaker wire. A pacemaker wire with failed insulation, may conduct a current into the heart and cause ventricular fibrillation.

Diathermy can be used if:
Bipolar where the current is concentrated across the tips of the forceps. Unipolar where the entry and exit points and the field of the current are more than 15 cm away from any part of the pacemaker circuit.

12. Pacemaker functions are written as five letters (NBG code).

- The chamber paced (A atrium V ventricle, D dual)
- The chamber sensed (AVD)
- The response to sensing (T triggered I inhibited D dual R reverse)
- Programmability
- Functions available in tachycardia.

VVI is: Ventricle paced, Ventricle sensed, response to sensing Inhibition.

Part II
1. $V = IR$.

2. $W = RI^2$ can be written as $P = IR^2$ where P = energy per unit time. Strictly $E = IR^2 \times T$.

3. Voltage 240, frequency 50 Hz. 50 Hz is the optimum current for causing ventricular fibrillation.

4. There are a number of means for protecting the patient from the mains electrical supply.
   a. Cut the current if there is excess by using:
      i. A fuse.
      ii. A current leakage detector, which warns or switches off the supply if the current passing in the neutral is not the same as in the earth lead.
      iii.A current-operated earth-leakage circuit breaker (ELCB) which detects the current in the live and the neutral which should be the same.
   b. Use an alternative power supply:
      i. A DC battery, this may be a dry cell or rechargeable.
      ii. An isolating transformer.
   c. Reduce the risk of current passing through the patient or staff to earth by
      i. An earth to the equipment casing.
      ii. Double insulation so the case is less likely to be alive.
   d. Ensure that the current passing through the patient is not at a dangerous frequency e.g. by using an isolating capacitor on the diathermy.

Answers – Self-test: Defibrillator

1. Broken earth connection on Apparatus. A leakage current can pass from the apparatus, to the patient and out through the electrodes because there is an earth through the monitor. The heating pad beneath the patient is broken so that a current can flow into the patient from this pad.

2. Micro-shock can occur with 1 volt, 150 microamps, if such a current passes through a catheter directly into the heart.

3. *a.* Microshock will cause ventricular fibrillation.
   b. Current applied to the skin below 1 milliamp is felt as a tingling, above this is it is felt as pain.
   c. A DC current will cause muscle contraction, an AC current muscle twitching.
   d. Skin burns at the point of contact.
   e. The heart will develop ectopic beats and ventricular fibrillation, particularly with AC current at 50 Hz supplied in UK. The risk of VF falls with high frequency current.

4. *A.* Read the instructions before use.
   B. On/Off switch.
   C. Type B equipment. Examples of this type of equipment either have no electrical contact with the patient, e.g. a pressure monitor on a breathing system, or is battery-operated, e.g. a nerve stimulator.
   D. Type BF equipment. Such equipment has an outer part earthed.
   E. Type CF equipment. Such equipment has an outer component, which is earthed, and an inner separate part, which is isolated from the mains connections. Less than 150 microamps can leak through the device. It is suitable for use when a defibrillator is attached, e.g. ECG monitor.
   F. Equipotentiality.

5. A – Peak potential of 5000 volts
   B – Capacitor
   C – Inductor
   D – Defibrillator pads.

6. A store of electrons equivalent to a charge of 35A × 4 ms = 140 m coulombs.

   There is a high initial current in the circuit, which dies away as the capacitor becomes charged.

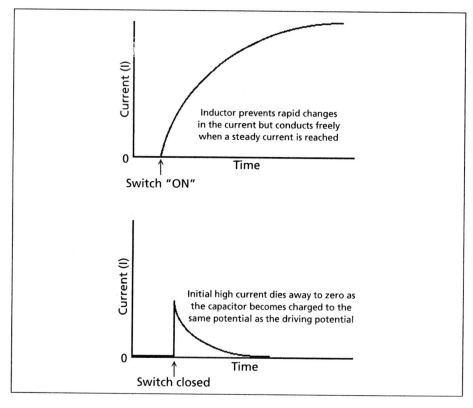

7. The inductor prolongs the duration of the flow of current. When the defibrillator is discharged the inductor absorbs some of the energy from the capacitor so not all is released to the patient. It prevents rapid changes in the current but conducts freely when a steady state is reached.

8. A coulomb is the flow of 1 ampere (A) for 1 second (s). This is 6.24 × 10¹⁸ electrons.

9. The stored energy depends on the voltage (V) and on the electrical charge (C = A × s).

   Power (W) = Potential (V) × Current (A).

   Power = Energy (J) per second.

   Coulombs are current (A) × seconds so:

   Energy (Joules) = Coulombs × Voltage.

   The stored energy is about half the peak potential.

   Stored energy = 1/2 × 5000 V × 35 A × 4 ms = 350 Joules.

10. The defibrillator delivers a current for a number of seconds. As the voltage drops, so the energy drops. The inductor is present to ensure that the output current has the best duration and waveform. It prolongs the duration of the flow of current. The inductor absorbs some of the energy stored in the capacitor. The output will be in the order of 35 amperes for a duration of 4–12 milliseconds.

11. The waveform is half a sinusoidal wave, duration 4–12 milliseconds.

12. The current causes simultaneous depolarisation of all cardiac muscle making the cells refractory to depolarisation.

13. The current should be synchronised to be applied about 20 milliseconds after the start of the R wave.

14. DC current is used because it is:
    a. more effective
    b. less myocardial damage
    c. less arrhythmogenic.

    The lower the energy the less the damage to the heart. An AC current cannot synchronise with the ECG.

15. Apply paddles to chest. One on the sternum and one on the left mid axillary line OR one paddle anterior over the left precordium and one posteriorly behind the heart. Firm pressure on the paddles:
    - Reduces the transthoracic impedance
    - Achieves a higher peak current flow.

    Take oxygen away, charge defibrillator, order stand clear and check obeyed, apply paddles firmly, apply shock, place paddles back on defibrillator, do not wave paddles in air.

16. The external paddles are 8–8.5 cm in diameter. Internal defibrillation depends on the size of the paddles and the size of the heart. An implanted automatic defibrillator monitors rhythm and applies a shock when a severe tachycardia is detected.

17. Skin burns and dysrhythmias.

SKILL

9

Skill 1   (Answers on page 277)

Try to complete all the questions. Have a guess if there is no negative marking on this station. You might come back to a question at the end if there is time.

You are asked to demonstrate how to assess a patient's airway.

Questions

1. Write down, in order, the features that you will check.

2. What might inspection show?

3. How far should the mouth open? What may limit opening?

4. The neck will normally move freely. Which condition may be associated with good movement but is a dangerous situation during intubation?

5. How can the shortness of the neck be assessed?

6. What is the Mallampati score? Describe exactly the grades.

7. What is the relationship between the Mallampati score and the Cormack and Lehane score?

8. Describe all the grades of the Cormack and Lehane score.

9. What is the significance of a history of snoring?

Skill 2

(Answers on page 278)

You are asked to demonstrate the technique of cricothyroid puncture on a neck manikin.

Questions

1. Demonstrate the correct position for the head.

2. Where is the needle introduced?

3. If oxygen is infused through a cannula without ventilating the lungs what will happen to the arterial carbon dioxide level?

4. Name at least two possible complications associated with cricothyroid puncture.

5. Is a percutaneous tracheostomy performed at the same site?

6. Name three indications for cricothyroid puncture.

7. At what depth will the cricothyroid membrane be punctured?

8. How would you deal with an obstruction to expiration once cricothyroid ventilation has been established?

9. Name one contraindication to cricothyroid puncture?

10. Label the anatomical structures on the diagram (opposite).

SAGITTAL SECTION OF THE NECK
(LABEL THE STRUCTURES MARKED ON THE DIAGRAM)

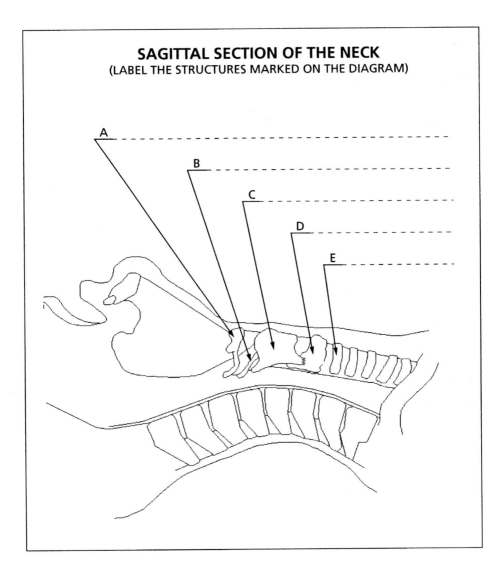

Skill 3

(Answers on page 279)

You are asked to demonstrate cricoid pressure on a manikin of the neck.

Questions

1. On the diagram opposite draw in the position of:

   - The thyroid cartilage.
   - The hyoid bone.
   - The trachea.
   - The internal jugular vein.
   - Sternomastoid and recurrent laryngeal nerves.

2. Which cartilage is pressure applied to?

3. What is the cartilage pressed against?

4. Which fingers are used?

5. How are the hands placed?

6. When should the pressure be removed?

7. When will this manoeuvre be less effective?

8. Who was Sellick?

9. What amount of pressure should be used?

10. What is the minimum time for satisfactory pre-oxygenation?

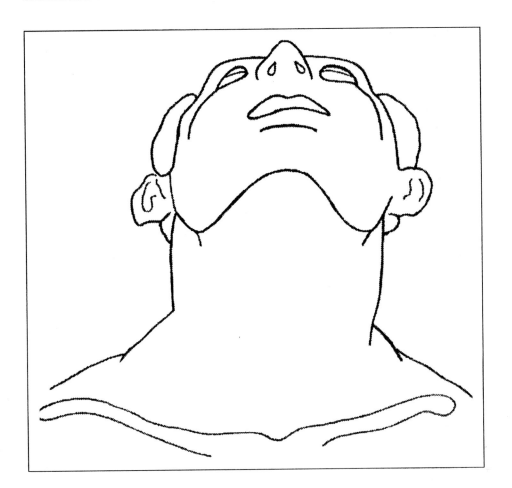

Skill 4

(Answers on page 280)

The diagram below includes a number of errors.

Questions

1. How many can you spot?

2. Draw lines to connect the apparatus to ensure a negative pressure on the drain of not more than 5 cm H_2O.

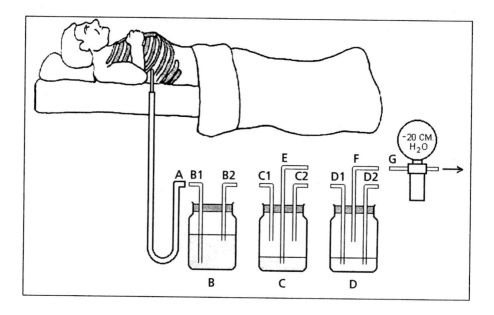

(Answers on page 281)

Skill 5

The diagram below includes a number of errors.

Questions
1. How many can you spot?

2. Is the pressure trace correct?

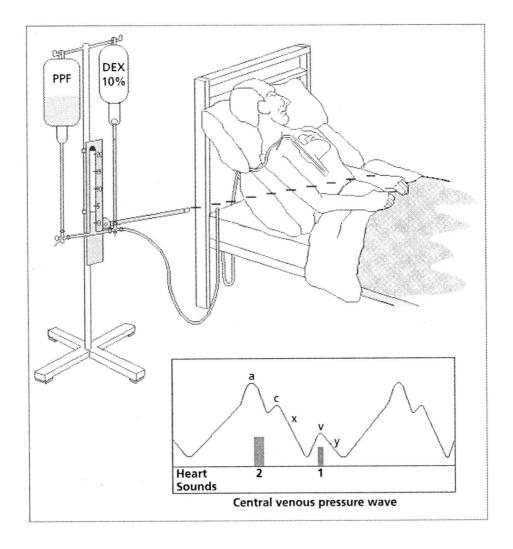

Central venous pressure wave

Skill 6

(Answers on page 282)

The diagram below includes a number of errors.

Question
1. How many can you spot?

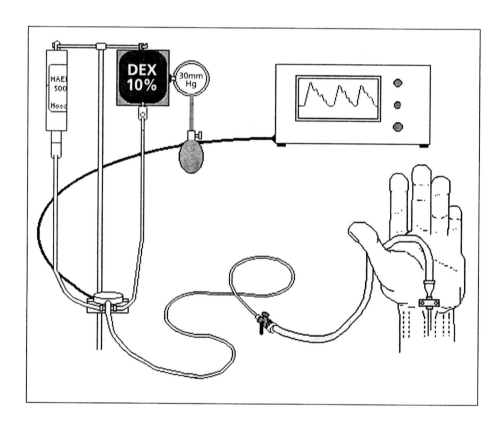

Three-in-one-block

Question

1. Label the diagram of the inguinal region (below). Describe the landmarks for identifying the point for injection to achieve a three-in-one block.

2. Which nerves should be blocked in performing a three-in-one block?

3. Which nerve roots do these nerves come from?

4. Name at least two situations for which three-in-one block might be relevant.

5. What volume of local anaesthetic is used?

6. What precautions are taken during injection of the local anaesthetic?

7. When using a nerve stimulator to locate the nerve:
   a. What current is supplied by the stimulator?
   b. Which are stimulated first as the current is increased, motor or sensory nerves?
   c. What current should be used so that the stimulus is not painful when applied directly to the nerve?
   d. Which pole of the stimulator should be applied to the nerve and which to the skin?

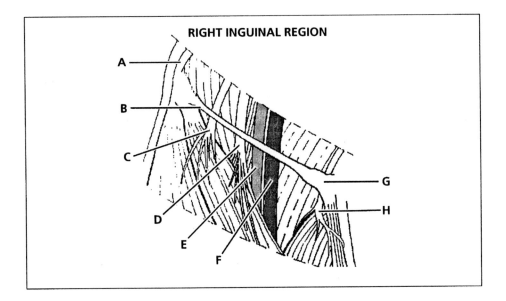

RIGHT INGUINAL REGION

Skill 8
(Answers on page 285)

Questions

1. Label the structures marked on the sagittal section of the spine shown opposite.

2. In the adult the spinal cord ends at the level of lumbar 3.   True   False

3. In adults the subarachnoid space ends at the level of lumbar 4.   True   False

4. The epidural space can be detected by using loss of resistance to air.   True   False

5. The depth from skin to epidural space is an average of about 4 cm.   True   False

6. The depth from skin to epidural space is further when the paramedian approach is used than when the midline approach is used.   True   False

7. The average total volume of each epidural space is 2 cc.   True   False

8. A test dose of 2 cc local anaesthetic at L2 will give a sensory blockade of the thighs if placed into the CSF.   True   False

9. The Tuohy needle is so named because it has a blunt end.   True   False

10. There is no epidural space inside the skull.   True   False

11. An epidural can be performed through the sacral hiatus.   True   False

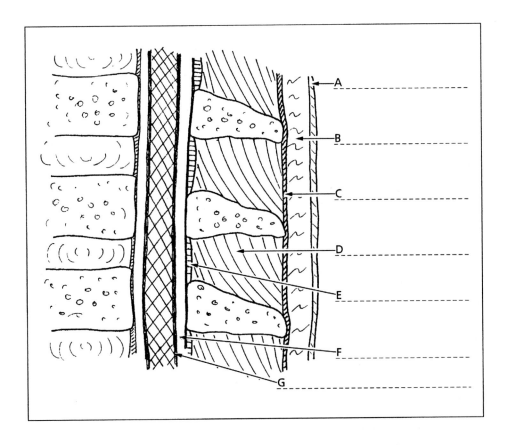

A _____

B _____

C _____

D _____

E _____

F _____

G _____

Skill 9

(Answers on page 286)

Local anaesthetic blocks for eye surgery.

Questions

1. What position should the eye be in for a periorbital nerve block and which position should be avoided?

2. Describe the first stage in the application of local anaesthetic.

3. What is the point of entry of the needle for a periorbital block?

4. How does a periorbital block differ from a retrobulbar block?

5. What is the furthest distance a needle should be introduced for a periorbital block?

6. Which muscle is supplied by the seventh cranial nerve and is blocked for eye surgery?

7. Name two complications of a periorbital block.

8. How would you diagnose and treat a retrobulbar haematoma?

9. Apart from 2% lignocaine and 0.75% bupivacaine what else might be included in a solution for periorbital block and why?

10. What are the features of a successful periorbital block?

(Answers on page 287)

Skill 10

Eye

Questions

1. Label the structures of the **eye** A to G.

2. Label the structures in and around the orbit A to F

3. Label the structures in the **right orbital fissure** that make up the ring around the optic nerve on the posterior wall of the orbit.

4. What do the following nerves supply?
   a. Third cranial nerve.
   b. Fourth cranial nerve.
   c. Sixth cranial nerve.

5. What is unusual about the sixth cranial nerve and what happens if its function is impaired?

6. Describe the mechanism for nystagmus.

7. Why does the pupil constrict when light is shone at it?

8. Which muscles control the position of the eyelids?

   You should be able to describe an eye block for a cataract operation.

9. What are the main problems concerning an eye block and how are they avoided.

10. What is the difference between a peribulbar and an intra-conal block?

11. How will you perform an eye block for a cataract extraction? Which approach will you use and why?

12. Trace the optic nerve from the back of the eye to the visual cortex.

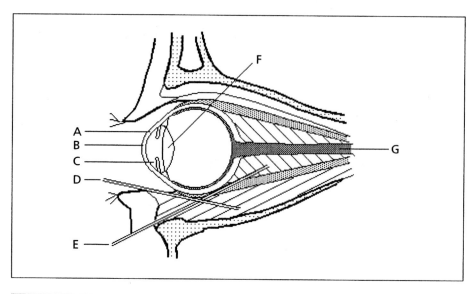

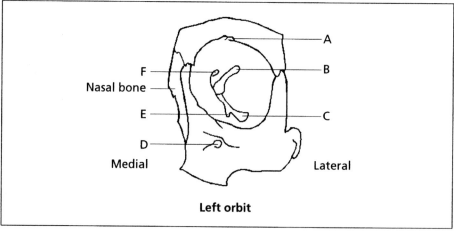

Left orbit

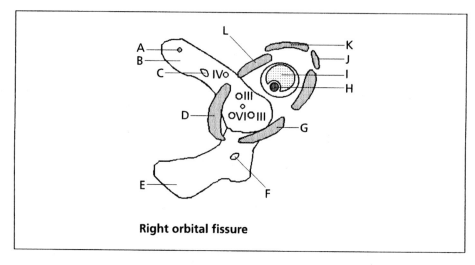

Right orbital fissure

(Answers on page 290)

Ankle block

Questions

1. Which cutaneous nerves cross the ankle?

2. Label A and B. How is this nerve blocked?

3. Label C and D. How is this nerve blocked?

4. Label E, F and G. How are these nerves blocked?

5. Label H, I and J. How is this nerve blocked?

6. What is the course of the saphenous nerve?

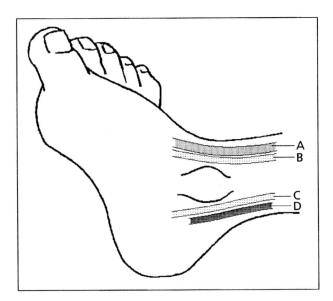

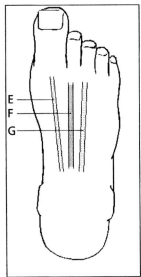

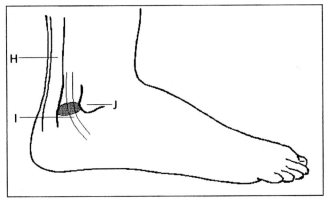

Answers
Skill

Answers – Skill 1

1, 2. General inspection. Visual appearance: obesity, facial scaring or deformity, cervical and thoracic spinal deformity, neck short or limited movement, mouth opening – prominent mandible or upper incisors.

Specific diseases: Rheumatoid arthritis, thoracic kyphosis, burns of the head and neck, congenital abnormality of head and neck.

3. Mouth opening: ask the patient to open their mouth. Can three or more fingers be inserted in the sagittal plane? Is movement of the tempero-mandibular joint limited?

4. Neck movement. Extension and flexion. A normal head should extend on the neck to at least 45° to the horizontal. Reduced movement may result from osteoarthritis, ankylosing spondylosis, rheumatoid arthritis and previous surgery. In rheumatoid arthritis an X-ray in extension and flexion for evidence of movement at the atlanto-occipital joint is essential to exclude subluxation.

5. Short neck: measure the thyro-mental distance with the head extended. Under 6 cm, or three finger widths, may be a problem for intubation.

6. Mallampati score.

Open the mouth and see the tonsillar fauces and pillars *score 1*. The uvula and upper fauces *score 2*. The soft palate and base of uvula *score 3*. The hard palate only (no soft palate visible) *score 4*. 3 and 4 may be a difficult intubation.

7. There is a correlation, but not an absolute one, between the two scores.

8. The score is: Total larynx seen *1*. Only the posterior larynx seen *2*. Epiglottis but no arytenoids seen *3*. No epiglottis seen *4*.

9. Snoring indicates a narrowing of some point in the airway when the muscles relax that support the airway between the sternum and the mandible. One site for obstruction is the tongue vibrating against the posterior pharyngeal wall or inlet to the larynx. This suggests there will be a poor view of the larynx at laryngoscopy due to the tongue or epiglottis blocking the view of the larynx. The patient will also be more prone to airway obstruction postoperatively.

Answers – Skill 2

1. The patient is supine with the neck extended.

2. The cricothyroid membrane – which connects the thyroid cartilage to the cricoid cartilage – is punctured anteriorly, in the mid line.

3. Arterial carbon dioxide will rise at the rate of 0.5 kPa (3 mmHg) every minute.

4. Complications include: puncturing the carotid artery, internal jugular vein, perforation of the oesophagus, pretracheal inflation of gas, barotrauma to the trachea, surgical emphysema in the neck as gas leaks back around the catheter puncture site, bronchial rupture and pneumothorax.

5. No. It involves puncturing the space between the first and second tracheal rings.

6. *a*. Emergency control of the airway.
   b. Topical anaesthesia of the larynx, e.g. for laryngospasm.
   c. Retrograde intubation of the larynx.
   d. Jet ventilation for laryngoscopy.
   e. Clearance of secretions following surgery, particularly thoracic surgery.

7. About 0.5 inches or 1 cm.

8. Try to relieve the obstruction by an oral airway, mouth suction or forward traction on the jaw. A second catheter may need to be introduced.

9. Trauma to the throat making it difficult to locate the landmarks. A large thyroid goitre or tumour obscuring the larynx.

10. A – Hyoid
    B – Epiglottic cartilage
    C – Thyroid cartilage
    D – Cricoid cartilage
    E – Trachea and tracheal ring.

Answers – Skill 3

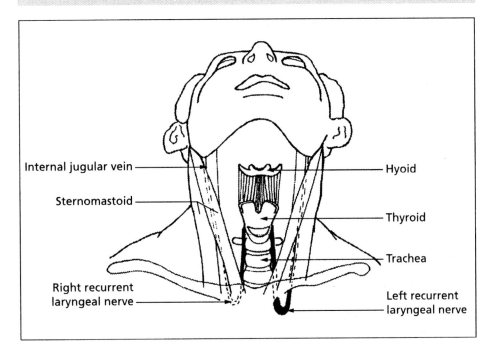

Internal jugular vein — Hyoid

Sternomastoid — Thyroid

— Trachea

Right recurrent laryngeal nerve — Left recurrent laryngeal nerve

1. As above.

2. The cricoid cartilage.

3. The body of the 6th cervical vertebra.

4. The thumb and middle finger are pressed onto the cartilage while the index finger is used to steady the mid-line.

5. One hand is used to press the cricoid cartilage while the other is placed behind the cervical spine. This is a bimanual manoeuvre.

6. Pressure is removed once the assistant has inflated the cuff or if the patient starts to vomit forcibly, to prevent rupture of the oesophagus.

7. In the presence of a nasogastric tube, a laryngeal mask and an oesophageal pouch. Once a laryngeal mask is in place it may be possible to apply cricoid pressure with effect but the presence of cricoid pressure may prevent the placement of the laryngeal mask.

8. A London anaesthetist who described the technique in the 1960s.

9. Up to 44 Newtons. This is equivalent to four 1 kg bags of sugar.

10. Adequate pre-oxygenation will occur in about 6 deep breaths which will replace the nitrogen in the lungs. It takes a further 3 minutes to replace most of the nitrogen in the rest of the body.

Answers – Skill 4

1. Wrong site to insert a catheter into the chest. Either 2nd space mid clavicular line or 4/5th space mid axillary line.

   Connecting tubing too long and draping on floor. Likely to increase the possibility of disconnection, kinking and the introduction of infection.

   The drainage bottles B,C, and D have no stoppers in the tops.

   The water depth in bottle B is too high, increasing the resistance to expanding the lung.

   The drainage tube B1 is too far into the water. This will increase the expiratory pressure and the pneumothorax may not expand.

   B2 should not be under the water.

   Bottle D is wrongly made up, C is correct. In D the tubes at the side are wrongly under the water while the centre tube is in free air. This will not produce a negative pressure.

2. To obtain about 5 cm H_2O – pipe B2 is connected to C1, then C2 connected to G and the suction turned on. The negative pressure is controlled by the depth of E under the water.

Answers – Skill 5

1. Wrong agents in the infusion bags. The solution used to make a reading should be normal saline, or Hartman's solution. 5% dextrose if there is concern about the conduction of an electric current.

   One administration set has no ball valve in the reservoir.

   One administration set reservoir is empty of fluid.

   No controllers on giving sets.

   No tap at bottom of measuring column.

   Sealed top to measuring column.

   Connecting tubing too long and draping on floor. Likely to cause damping and will increase possibility of disconnection, kinking and introducing infection.

   Catheter tip in inferior vena cava and not at entry to right atrium.

   The reading as drawn is below zero and is not physiologically possible, unless the patient breathes in against a resistance to create a marked negative intra-thoracic pressure. The reading is not compatible with a venous return sustaining a cardiac output. The patient should ideally be flat if an accurate reading is being made.

2. The a,c,v trace relating to the heart sounds is not correctly labelled. The a wave should be lined up with the first heart sound. The second heart sound occurs with the v wave. The x descent is between the a and c waves, during atrial relaxation. The y descent is between the c and the v wave, during atrial emptying.

Answers – Skill 6

1. The fluids for infusion are wrong. There should only be one isotonic crystalloid, such as saline, to infuse into the artery.

   The pressure in the surrounding bag is too low. It should be at least 50% above systolic pressure. There is no pressure bag on the gelatin line which runs directly to the arterial line.

   There is no clamp on the giving sets.

   There is no fluid in one of the reservoir chambers.

   There is no ball valve in one chamber.

   The tubing between the transducer and the patient is too long, and too wide.

   There is no tap near to the patient from which to sample arterial blood or to flush the line.

   There is no obvious continuous flushing device.

   The pressure trace shows resonance.

   The cannula should enter the wrist between abductor pollucis longus and flexor carpi radialis (FCR). Not FCR and palmaris longus.

Answers – Skill 7

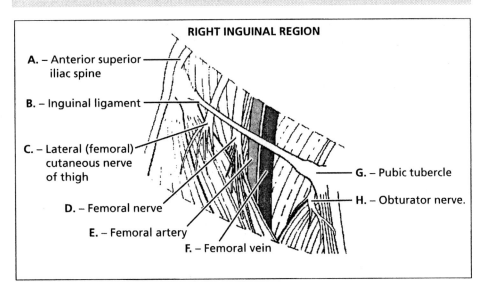

RIGHT INGUINAL REGION

A. – Anterior superior iliac spine

B. – Inguinal ligament

C. – Lateral (femoral) cutaneous nerve of thigh

D. – Femoral nerve

E. – Femoral artery

F. – Femoral vein

G. – Pubic tubercle

H. – Obturator nerve.

1. A–H as above.

   Palpate the anterior superior iliac spine and the pubic tubercle. Mark the inguinal ligament which joins these two points. Mark the mid point of this line which should be the point at which the femoral artery can be felt pulsating. The femoral nerve lies about 1 cm or a finger's width lateral to the artery. A short bevelled needle is introduced over the nerve and below the inguinal ligament. Pulsation of the artery may be felt as the needle is advanced. Paraesthesia will be obtained when the needle is near the nerve at a depth of about 3–4 cm.

2. Femoral, lateral (femoral) cutaneous nerve of the thigh and obturator nerves.

3. The anterior primary rami of lumbar 2, 3 and 4 which form the lumbar plexus.

4. Pain relief following operations on the knee, shaft and neck of femur, skin grafts from the thigh.

5. 20 ml was originally recommended and is suitable for a femoral block. 30 ml is used for a three-in-one block.

6. Monitor for intravascular injection. Apply pressure over the femoral nerve distal to the point of injection to encourage proximal spread of the local anaesthetic.

7. **a.** 6–8 volts limited to 30 milliamps. The impulse is 0.3 millisecond or less, duration at 2 Hz or 50 Hz.
   b. Motor nerves are stimulated first at 2 Hz. Sensory nerves are stimulated at 50 Hz. High frequencies (50 Hz) produce pain before lower frequencies (2 Hz).

c. 2 Hz or 50 Hz and under 0.5 milliamp.

d. The negative is applied to the nerve as there is a greater density of current around the negative and so about 30% less current is required to produce a stimulus. It also helps to localise the nerve more accurately.

Answers – Skill 8

1. **A** – Skin
   B – Subcutaneous tissue
   C – Supraspinous ligament
   D – Interspinous ligament
   E – Ligamentum flavum
   F – Epidural space
   G – Dura mater.

2. **False** – The subarachnoid space extends to the sacrum in the foetus. Due to the bone growing faster than the nerve tissue of the cord the cord finishes at about lumbar 1 in the adult.

3. **False** – The subarachnoid finishes at sacral 1, below which the dura continues as the filum terminale.

4. **True** – The space can be detected by loss of resistance to air or fluid, or the negative pressure in the lumbar region.

5. **True** – The normal range is 3–5 cm.

6. **True.**

7. **False** – The average volume is 4 cc; greater in the sacral region. The space is occupied by nerve roots, vessels and adipose tissue, so this is not the volume of local anaesthetic required to fill the space.

8. **True** – The thigh is innervated by L1, 2, 3 nerve roots.

9. **False** – The blunt end is the Huber point. The side opening is the Tuohy needle.

10. **True** – The epidural space ends at the foramen magnum and is only a potential space inside the skull.

11. **True** – The sacral hiatus is where the spine of S5 might have been and is a portal into the sacral canal.

Answers – Skill 9

1. The patient should look straight ahead. In the past the patient might have looked up and medially for a retrobulbar block. This brings the optic nerve and vessels into prominence and into a position where they are more likely to be punctured.

2. The conjunctiva and cornea are anaesthetised with 4% lignocaine, amethocaine 0.5% or oxybuprocaine 0.4% eye drops. Cocaine is avoided as it may damage the cornea. In order to reduce patient discomfort, a series of instillations are made starting with a dilute solution.

3. At the inferior-lateral angle of the eye through the conjunctiva. A second point may be used: through the conjunctiva between the superior orbital notch and the medial canthus.

4. **a.** The retrobulbar block needle is usually introduced through the skin of the eyelid and pierces the muscle cone.
   b. The periorbital block needle enters through the conjunctiva and stays outside the muscle cone.

5. 25 mm.

6. The orbicularis oculi is blocked to prevent involuntary blinking. If the seventh nerve is not blocked in the orbit a separate block can be made. Part of the nerve can be blocked outside the lateral margin of the orbit in the temporal area or all the nerve is blocked in front of the tragus in the parotid area.

7. Vasovagal reaction, haematoma, total spinal with local anaesthetic entering the CSF and intravascular effects of local anaesthetic.

8. The eye becomes tense and pushes forward. Apply pressure for 20–30 minutes, delay surgery and possibly perform a canthotomy.

9. Hyaluronidase 500 units/5 ml to encourage spread of the local anaesthetic and possibly reduce intra ocular pressure. Adrenaline or other vasoconstrictor to reduce bleeding and prolong the effect of the block and orbital akinesia.

10. Anaesthesia of the eye, a dilated pupil, exophthalmos, reduced intra ocular pressure and an immobile eye.

Answers – Skill 10

1. **A** – Angle of Schlemm from which the aqueous humour is absorbed.
   B – Cornea
   C – Iris
   D – Needle for peribulbar block
   E – Needle for retrobulbar block
   F – Lens
   G – Optic nerve.

2. **A** – Supra orbital notch
   B – Superior orbital fissure
   C – Inferior orbital fissure
   D – Infra-orbital foramen
   E – Infra-orbital groove
   F – Optic canal.

3. **A** – Lacrimal nerve
   B – Superior orbital fissure
   C – Frontal nerve and superior ophthalmic vein
   D – Lateral rectus
   E – Inferior orbital fissure
   F – Inferior ophthalmic vein
   G – Inferior rectus
   H – Ophthalmic artery
   I – Optic nerve
   J – Superior oblique with medial rectus below and lateral
   K – Levator palpebrae superioris
   L – Superior rectus.

4. ▪ Third nerve supplies, medial, superior and inferior recti and inferior oblique.
   ▪ Fourth nerve supplies superior oblique.
   ▪ Sixth nerve supplies lateral rectus (LR_6SO_4).

5. The sixth cranial nerve has the longest intracranial course of all cranial nerves. Reduced function is associated with a failure to move the eye laterally. The patient notices a double vision. The sixth cranial nerve function is affected after illness, surgery and anaesthesia, tiredness. It recovers fully without treatment.

6. Nystagmus is caused by drifting of the eyes from a point of fixation towards a position of rest with a rapid correction back to the point of fixation. It is not a disorder of the eye but of the cerebellum.

7. The light impulse is sensed by the retina and travels along the optic nerve and optic tract to the Edringer–Westphal nucleus. From here preganglionic fibres go to the ciliary ganglion through the oculomotor nerve. The postganglionic fibres travel with the short ciliary nerves to the

sphincter pupillae muscle. The reflex is bilateral as nerves in the optic tract go to both nuclei.

8. The levator palpebrae superioris raises open the upper lid and orbicularis oculi closes both lids together.

9. **a.** The eye punctured by the needle. A blunt needle will reduce this possibility but is painful to inject. The eye ball should not move when the needle is moved. A sharp needle is easier to inject and is unlikely to pierce the sclera, which is very thick, without force.

   b. Optic nerve damage. If the needle is not injected behind the eye then it will not reach the optic nerve. The eyeball is usually 20–25 mm long except in the myopic eye when it is longer. If the needle is injected less than 25 mm from the front of the eye it is not retrobulbar.

   c. Intravascular injection and injection into the subarachnoid space require immediate resuscitation.

   d. Haematoma is a lesser problem, which is usually controlled by gentle pressure.

   e. Conjunctival oedema.

   f. Corneal abrasion.

   g. Myopathy of extraocular muscles.

   h. Vaso-vagal attack, commoner in children squint surgery and stimulation of medial rectus.

   Mechanism. Traction on the extraocular muscles, especially the medial rectus creates nerve impulses in the short and long ciliary nerves – ophthalmic branch of the trigeminal nerve – Gasserian ganglion in the reticular formation. In the reticular formation from the sensory trigeminal nucleus to the motor nucleus of the vagus – vagus nerve to the SA node.

10. A peribulbar block lies around the orbit. The needle is inserted no more than the long axis or length of the eye (20–25 mm). A retrobulbar block is behind the orbit; i.e. the needle is in more than 25 mm. The needle may lie outside the cone and so away from the optic nerve (or intraconal) and so nearer to the optic nerve. The diagram shows both needles retrobulbar, one is outside the cone while the other is inside the cone.

11. Have it clear in your mind – are you describing a periorbital block when the needle is no deeper than the long axis of the eye. A retrobulbar block when the needle is past the posterio border of the eye which is either intraconal or extraconal.

The inferior lateral approach has the advantage that the optic nerve is medial in the orbit so a long way from the needle. There is often a gap in the cone of muscles inferior lateral and LA given peribulbar can pass in to the cone with quicker onset of action as all the sensory nerves are within the cone. The superior medical approach is near to the optic nerve and the needle should only be introduced to 10–12 mm.

All the equipment for resuscitation. Explanation to patient, consent.

The patient lies looking straight ahead. Increasing concentrations of LA are place on the conjunctiva to make a painless cornea block. A blunt or sharp 25 G needle is introduced at the lower lateral angle of the conjunctiva for less than 25 mm from the front of the eye. The eye should not move when the needle is moved. No resistance to passage of needle, aspirate. Inject 3–7 ml, 2% lidocaine or equivalent with hyaluronidase 500 units.

12. The optic nerve runs for 12.5 mm from the back of the globe of the eye to the optic foramen within the muscle cone.

    The two optic nerves pass medial to the internal carotid artery, then join and divide in the optic chiasma around the pituitary. The fibres carrying sensation from the nasal fields stay on the same side. The fibres carrying temporal sensations cross over to the other side. A pituitary enlargement presses on the crossing fibres first to give a bitemporal field defect.

    The tracts pass to the lateral geniculate body, to the optic radiation and then to the visual cortex.

Answers – Skill 11

1. There are five nerves at the ankle:
   - Saphenous
   - Tibial
   - Deep peroneal
   - Superficial peroneal nerve
   - Sural nerve.

2. **A** – Saphenous vein
   B – Saphenous nerve.

   Saphenous nerve lies:
   Anterior to the medial malleolus but posterior to the long saphenous vein.

   Injection 1 cm anterior and proximal to the medial malleolus. 5 ml LA subcutaneously.

3. **C** – Tibial nerve
   D – Tibial artery.

   Landmarks:
   Behind the medial malleolus but anterior to the tibial artery pulsation.

   Injection palpate the posterior tibial artery and leave a finger on the artery. Inject anterior to the artery, behind the medial malleolus pointing towards the artery.

4.
   E – Deep peroneal nerve
   F – Dorsalis pedis artery
   G – Superficial peroneal nerve.

   Deep peroneal nerve lies on the dorsum of the ankle/foot.

   Dorsalis pedis artery lies at the mid point of a line between the malleoli and runs to the first web space. The nerve lies on the medial side of the artery.

   Inject 1 cm medial to the artery.

   Superficial peroneal nerve lies lateral to the dorsalis pedis pulsation.

   Inject 7 ml subcutaneously across the dorsum of the ankle.

5.
   H – Achilles tendon
   I – Sural nerve
   J – Lateral malleolus.

   Sural nerve lies posterior to the lateral malleolus but anterior to Achilles tendon.

   Infiltrate 5 ml between malleolus and tendon.

6. Saphenous nerve is the longest cutaneous branch of the femoral nerve.

Arises from the posterior division, in the femoral triangle, descends lateral to the femoral artery. In the adductor canal crosses in front of the femoral artery to lie on its medial side. Between sartorius and gracilis to the medial border of the tibia behind the saphenous vein and then in front of the medial malleolus.

ANATOMY 10

Anatomy 1 *(Answers on page 313)*

Skull face

Questions

1. On the diagram (below), what are the structures and lines labelled A to F?

2. Which nerves leave through these foramen?

3. What is the significance of each facial fracture?

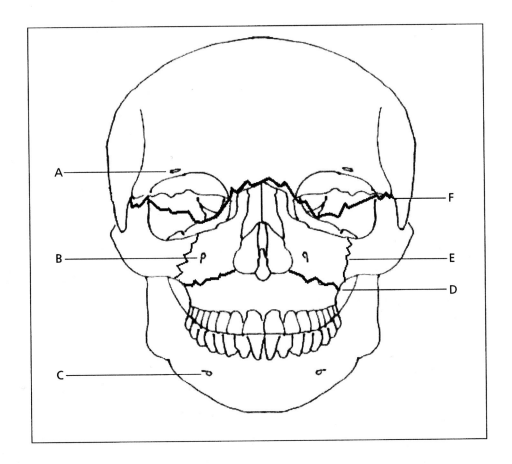

Anatomy 2
(Answers on page 315)

Base of skull

The skull has clinical importance in nerve blocks, particularly peribulbar and trigeminal blocks, jugular venous bulb sampling and intracranial pressure measurement. The important structures are in italics.

The following are the important foramen on the base of the skull, with the structures that are related or pass through them.

Cribriform plate
- *Olfactory nerve*
- *Covered by meninges containing the CSF*
- *Anterior and posterior ethmoidal arteries and nerves*

Optic canal
- *Optic nerve passing to the superior orbital foramen*
- Ophthalmic artery
- Meninges

Foramen spinosum
- *Middle meningeal artery*
- Meningeal branch of mandibular nerve
- Zygomatic branch of the facial nerve.

Foramen ovale
- *Mandibular branch of trigeminal nerve*
- Accessory meningeal artery

Foramen rotundum
- *Maxillary branch of trigeminal nerve*

Foramen lacerum
- Internal carotid artery pierces the posterior wall and ascends in its upper part.

Jugular foramen from forwards to behind
- Inferior petrosal sinus
- *Glossopharyngeal nerve IX, vagus nerve X, accessory nerve XI*
- *Sigmoid sinus, continuous with the internal jugular vein*

Hypoglossal canal
- Hypoglossal nerve

Foramen magnum
- *Spinal cord, lower part of the medulla*
- Spinal artery
- Vertebral artery

Carotid canal
- *Internal carotid artery*

Stylomastoid foramen
- Facial nerve
- Stylomastoid branch of posterior auricular artery.

Internal auditory meatus
- Facial nerve, motor and sensory
- Vestibulocochlear nerve
- Labyrinthine vessels

Questions

1. Label the features indicated on the base of skull picture by A–G.

2. Air and odours penetrate the cribriform plate. True False

3. The carotid artery passes through the foramen lacerum. True False

4. The fourth cranial nerve passes through the foramen rotundum. True False

5. The mandibular nerve passes through the foramen ovale. True False

6. The maxillary nerve passes through the foramen spinosum. True False

7. Behind and lateral to the foramen lacerum on the base of the skull is a depression. This is filled by the gasserian ganglion. True False

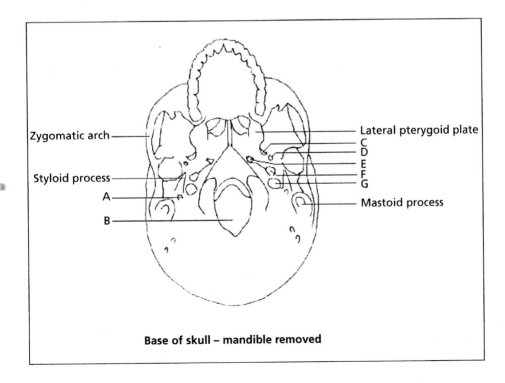

Zygomatic arch

Lateral pterygoid plate
C
D
E
Styloid process
F
G

A

Mastoid process

B

Base of skull – mandible removed

8. The 9, 10 and 11 cranial nerves pass through the jugular foramen?   True   False

9. An acoustic neuroma is likely to grow at the internal acoustic meatus.   True   False

10. The effects of such a neuroma include difficulty in swallowing.   True   False

11. An adult has 28 teeth when all are present.   True   False

12. The carotid artery occupies the carotid canal.   True   False

13. Local anaesthetic at the foramen ovale will cause numbness of the lower teeth.   True   False

14. The following structures pass though the foramen magnum.
Meninges, vertebral arteries, roots of accessory nerve, extradural space.   True   False

(Answers on page 316)

The vagus nerve

Questions

1. Label the nuclei of the vagus nerve and associated tracts in this cross-section of the medulla oblongata.

2. What are the names and functions of the vagal nuclei?

3. What is the course and relationships of the vagus nerve in the neck?

4. What is the course of the right vagus below the neck?

5. What is the course of the left vagus below the neck?

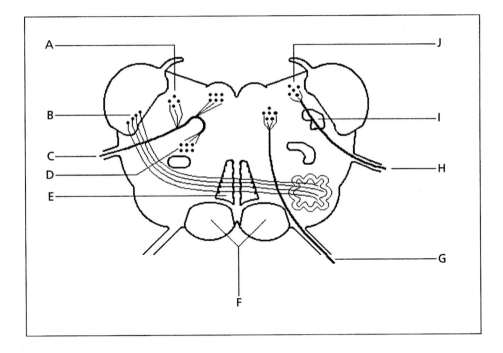

Anatomy 4 (Answers on page 318)

The sympathetic nervous system

Questions

1. Describe the efferent sympathetic pathway from the brain to an end organ in the head, heart or leg.

2. *a.* Where is the coeliac plexus sited?
   b. Label the structures on the diagram and the CT scan and draw in the coeliac plexus with the needle position for a coeliac block.
   c. What is the problem that might make a coeliac block difficult on the CT scan?

3. Which nerves synapse or pass through plexus?

4. What are the steps in performing a coeliac plexus block?

5. What are the complications of coeliac block?

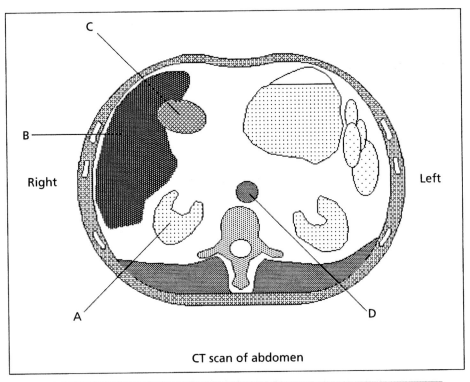

CT scan of abdomen

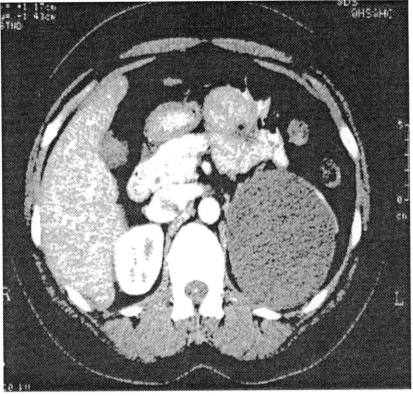

Anatomy 5

(Answers on page 320)

Stellate ganglion block

Questions

1. What is the stellate ganglion?

2. What are the relationships of the stellate ganglion?

3. What is the effect of blocking the stellate ganglion?

4. When might a stellate ganglion block be used in clinical practice?

5. How would you perform a stellate ganglion block?

6. What are the complications of performing this block?

Anatomy 6 (Answers on page 321)

Spinal cord

Questions

1. Label the structures A to I on the cross-section of the spinal cord.

2. What is the length of the spinal cord?

3. What is the origin and end of the spinal cord?

4. The spinal cord is made up of grey and white matter. Describe the grey matter.

5. Describe the white matter.

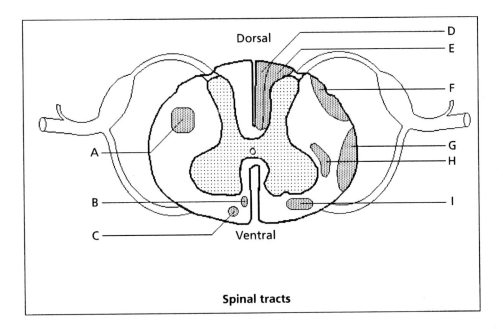

Anatomy 7

(Answers on page 323)

Arterial blood supply to the brain

Questions

1. In the top figure opposite, label the arteries on the base of the brain.

2. Which arteries supply the circle of Willis?

3. What are the branches of the carotid artery in the cranium?

4. In the bottom figure opposite, label the vessels on the section of the cord. What is important about the area E? Describe the blood supply to the cord.

5. What is the spinal artery syndrome?

6. What happens in transection of the cord?

7. What are the differences between CSF and plasma?

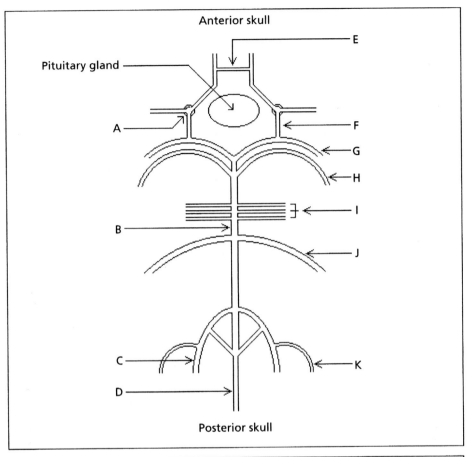

Anterior skull

Pituitary gland

E

A

F

G

H

I

B

J

C

K

D

Posterior skull

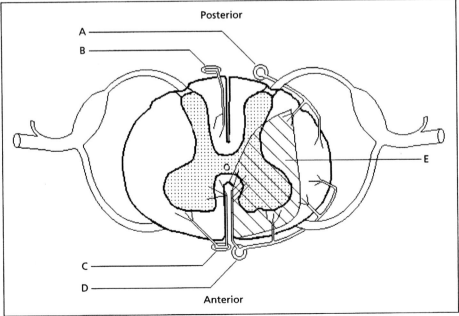

Posterior

A

B

E

C

D

Anterior

Anatomy 8
(Answers on page 326)

The coronary circulation

Questions

1. Name the structures A to E in the top diagram opposite.

2. What condition will occur if there is an acute, complete occlusion of artery A?

3. How would this be diagnosed?

4. How would you diagnose an acute blockage at C?

5. What is the Thesbian circulation?

6. What percentage of cardiac output does not drain into the coronary sinus?

7. What is the significance of the Thesbian circulation?

8. What other vessels contribute to this effect?

9. What is the nerve supply to the myocardium?

10. What is the ejection fraction?

11. How is the ejection fraction determined?

12. At the bottom of the opposite page, what are the vessels shown on the coronary arteriogram? On the diagram, what do 1 – MS, 2 – LC and 3 – LAD represent?

13. What are the origins of the left and right coronary arteries? What is the venous drainage of the heart?

What is the conducting system of the heart?

14. Where is the sinuatrial node?

15. Where is the atrioventricular node?

16. What is the blood supply of these nodes and the conducting system?

17. What are the layers of the heart?

18. How many cusps do the heart valves have and what prevents the valves being pushed backwards when under pressure? What are the sinuses of Valsalva?

19. What is the significance of the septomarginal trabecula (moderator band)?

20. What is the main venous drainage of the heart?

21. What is the blood oxygen saturation in the coronary sinus?

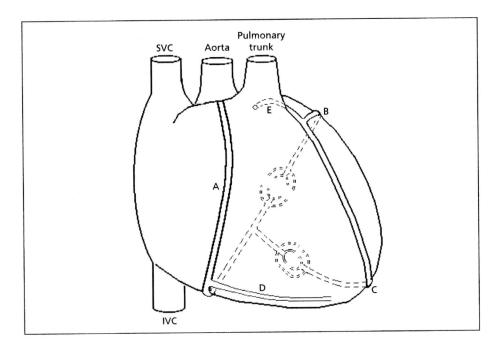

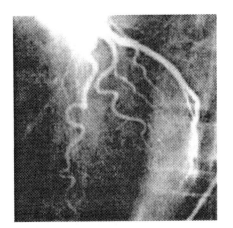

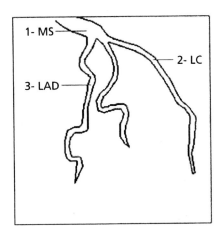

Left anterior oblique view

Anatomy 9 *(Answers on page 329)*

Brachial plexus block

Questions

1. What does this diagram represent?

2. Which nerve roots 1 to 5 make up this structure?

3. Name the labelled nerves A to G.

4. Name the relationships of the plexus above the clavicle.

5. What are the main landmarks for performing:
   a. an interscalene block
   b. a supraclavicular block
   c. an axillary block.

6. Which arm nerves can be missed when making an axillary block?

7. Which two major branches of the plexus are most readily blocked by the axillary approach?

8. Describe the axillary approach for a brachial plexus block and the problems that may arise.

9. Describe the interscalene approach.

10. What are the problems and complications of this block?

11. Describe the supraclavicular approach to the brachial plexus. How is this different from the subclavian, perivascular block?

12. What complications may arise from this block?

13. What are the maximum doses of local anaesthetic that should not be exceeded?

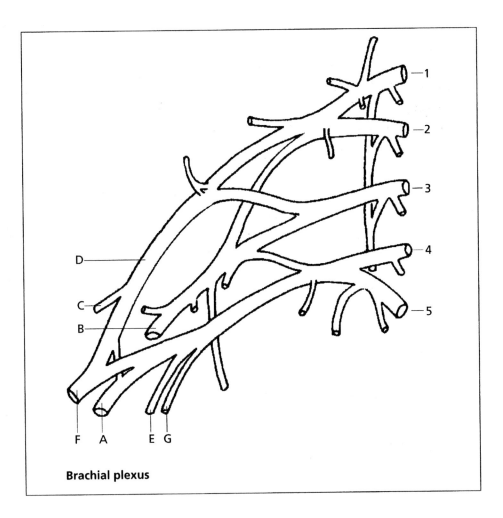

Brachial plexus

Anatomy 10 *(Answers on page 332)*

Nerves of the lower limb

Questions

1. Which anterior primary rami supply the lower limb?

2. What are the main plexuses and nerves to the lower limb?

(Answers on page 334)

Antecubital fossa

Anatomy of the antecubital fossa has the following relevance:

- How to insert central access peripherally and associated problems.
- How to check superficial and deep arterial system in hand.
- How you would perform median nerve block.
- How you would perform ulnar nerve block.
- Relative anatomy of the brachial artery.

Questions

1. Label the parts A to H of the antecubital fossa and the biceps tendon.

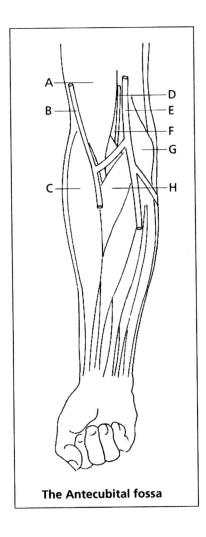

The Antecubital fossa

2. The shaded areas of the hands show the sensory distribution of which nerves?

3. What are the main groups of veins draining the upper limb?

4. What are the named superficial veins of the upper limb and their relationships?

5. What are the deep veins of the arm and their relationships?

6. Describe the important relationships of the radial nerve in the arm.

7. What is the course of the brachial artery?

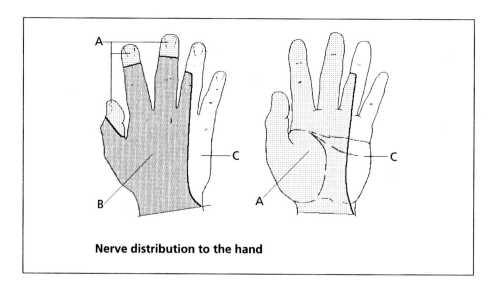

Nerve distribution to the hand

(Answers on page 336)

Wrist

The anatomy of the wrist is important for:

Local anaesthetics, stimulation of the nerves to assess neuromuscular blockade and arterial cannulation.

Questions

1. Label the structures on the diagram A to F.

Draw the position of the ulnar nerve and abductor pollucis

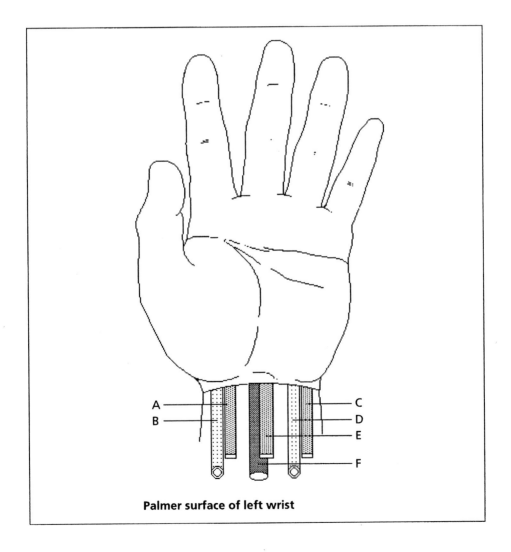

Palmer surface of left wrist

Answers
Anatomy

Answers – Anatomy 1

1. **A** – Supra-orbital foramen.
   B – Infra-orbital foramen.
   C – Mental nerve.
   D – Le Fort I fracture.
   E – Le Fort II fracture.
   F – Le Fort III fracture.

2. **A.** Supra-orbital nerve from the ophthalmic division of the trigeminal nerve. Carries unilateral sensation from the forehead as far as the crown except for a small area in the mid line, supplied by the supratrochlear nerve. Also sensation from the tip of the nose,
   B. Infra-orbital nerve from the maxillary division of the trigeminal nerve. Carries sensation from the cheek and upper lip.
   C. Mental nerve from the mandibular division of the trigeminal nerve. Carries sensation from over the mandible and the chin.

3. The fractures of the face are:
   a. Mandible fractures
   - Unilateral is usually stable.
   - Bilateral gives a floating central portion.
   Problems include, lacerations and bleeding inside the mouth, loose teeth and debris, oedema and swelling of the tongue and other soft tissues of the oropharynx.
   b. Le Fort fractures type I, II and III
   - Le Fort I is a horizontal fracture of the lower maxilla leading to a mobile palate.
   - Le Fort II is type I with oblique fractures along the malar-maxillary suture into the floor of the orbit. The maxilla is displaced backwards and free floating.
   - Type III is a transverse fracture of the face above the malar bones, through the orbit. This fracture separates the maxilla from the cranium. The face looks dish-like.

Type II and III fractures lead to nasal trauma and epistaxis, dural tears and CSF leaks. Nasal intubation (and naso-gastric tubes) should be avoided as it will lead to more trauma of the nasal passage, even penetrating the cribriform plate. **Only use oral tubes.**

If a difficult intubation is anticipated an inhalation induction should be performed or an oral fibreoptic laryngoscopy. LA may not work very well because of the trauma and blood on the mucus membranes.

The fractured mandible will usually move easily forward. If the hyoid is also damaged the hyo-epiglottic ligament may not raise the epiglottis so it is necessary to lift the epiglottis with a Magill, straight blade, type laryngoscope.

Answers – Anatomy 2

1. *A.* Stylomastoid foramen
   B. Foramen magnum
   C. Foramen ovale
   D. Foramen spinosum
   E. Foramen lacerum
   F. Carotid canal
   G. Jugular foramen

2. **False** – The olfactory nerves.

3. **True** – Internal carotid artery.

4. **False** – Maxillary division of trigeminal nerve.

5. **True** – Mandibular division of trigeminal nerve and accessory meningeal artery.

6. **False** – Middle meningeal artery and meningeal branch of mandibular nerve.

7. **True** – The ganglion of the trigeminal nerve lies in the Cave of Retzius.

8. **True** – Also the sigmoid sinus leading to the internal jugular vein; accessory, vagus and glossopharyngeal nerves; anteriorly the inferior petrosal sinus.

9. **True** – In the region of the internal acoustic meatus.

10. **False** – 8th nerve pressure leads to deafness. 7th nerve pressure leads to facial weakness.

11. **False** – 32.

12. **True** – Internal carotid artery.

13. **True** – Block of mandibular division of trigeminal nerve.

14. **False** – All pass except the extradural space.

Answers – Anatomy 3

1. **A** – Tractus solitarus.
   B – Olivo-cerebellar tact.
   C – IX and X nerve roots.
   D – Nucleus ambiguus.
   E – Medial meniscus.
   F – Pyramids.
   G – XII nerve root.
   H – X nerve root.
   I – Spinal tract of V.
   J – Dorsal nucleus.

   The vagus nerve is the longest, most widely distributed cranial nerve. The name means the wanderer. It carries motor, sensory and secretomotor nerves.

   Motor to: larynx, bronchial muscles, GIT as far as the splenic flexure, heart cardio-inhibitory.

   Sensory from: dura, external auditory meatus, respiratory tract, alimentary tract as far as the ascending colon, heart, epiglottis (gustatory).

   Secretomotor.

   Bronchial mucus glands, GIT.

2. Three vagal nuclei:
   a. Dorsal nucleus: mixed motor and sensory. Situated below the floor of the 4th ventricle.
   b. Nucleus ambiguus: motor nucleus. Situated within the reticular formation of the medulla.
   c. Tractus solitarus: sensation of taste. Situated in the grey matter of the medulla.

3. The vagus emerges for the medulla lateral to the Olive. It leaves the skull though the jugular foramen. At the base of the skull there are two ganglia:
   - Inferior sensory
   - Superior sensory.

   Below the inferior ganglion there is a communication with the accessory nerve.

   The nerve descends through the neck in the carotid sheath, between the carotid artery and jugular vein, into the thorax. The sympathetic trunk lies behind the carotid sheath.

4. From the root of the neck the right vagus crosses the first part of the subclavian artery.

   It gives off the recurrent laryngeal nerve at the lower border of this artery then passes behind the right brachio-cephalic vein.

In the thorax
The nerve descends into the thorax against the lateral aspect of the trachea. It is crossed by the azygos vein. It is separated from the lung only by the pleura. Behind the root of the lung it forms the right posterior pulmonary plexus sending branches into the lung and to the posterior oesophageal plexus.

In the abdomen, the right (posterior) vagus passes through the oesophageal hiatus in the diaphragm to the right and behind the oesophagus. It gives branches to the stomach and a large coeliac branch to the coeliac ganglion, which innervates the kidney, adrenals and intestine.

5. Left vagus enters the thorax between the carotid artery and the subclavian artery behind the left brachio-cephalic vein.

   Crosses the arch of the aorta near where the phrenic nerve passes over the aorta.

   At the lower border of the aortic arch the recurrent laryngeal nerve is given off and loops back around the aorta or the remnant of the ductus arteriosus into the neck.

   The main nerve passes behind the lung root and divides into the posterior pulmonary plexus. From this plexus branches descend on the front of the oesophagus to form an anterior oesophageal plexus.

In the abdomen
The left vagus passes through the oesophageal hiatus in the diaphragm in front of the oesophagus.

Branches to the cardia, stomach and a large hepatic nerve.

Answers – Anatomy 4

1. Efferent sympathetic pathways come from the posterior hypothalamus (parasympathetic fibres from anterior and tubular parts). The frontal lobe has an inhibitory effect on these centres. These efferent fibres pass to the mammillary body of the thalamus, then to the cingulate gyrus descending in lateral and anterior columns of the spinal cord to synapse with preganglionic cells in the lateral horn of the thoracic and upper lumbar cord.

   The grey H in the thoracic region is characterised by the lateral horn.

   Preganglionic, myelinated fibres leave the lateral horn with the ventral ramus. Almost at once they leave the ventral ramus to enter a sympathetic ganglion. One ganglion is associated with each spinal nerve below T1. In the neck there is an upper, middle and inferior ganglion (the inferior combines with T1 to form a stellate ganglion). In the ganglion, the nerves either synapse with a postganglionic, unmyelinated fibre or pass through to another ganglia at another level.

   The postganglionic fibres rejoin the anterior ramus through a grey ramus to be distributed with the nerves, except in the head and neck where the sympathetic nerves run with the arterial vessels.

   The sympathetic trunk is made up of two lines of ganglia lying on the cervical transverse processes, the head of the ribs in the thoracic region, anterio-lateral to the lumbar vertebrae and on the sacrum, from the skull to the coccyx.

   Key points
   - The stellate ganglion is the final path to the head, neck and upper arm.
   - The coeliac plexus is the common pathway for all sympathetic nerves from below the abdomen to enter the spinal cord.
   - Cardiac accelerator nerves originate at T2 to 4.

2. *a.* The coeliac plexus is retroperitoneal, surrounding the root of the coeliac artery, which lies at the superior border of the pancreas on a level with L1 vertebra.

   Relations anterior to T12 and L1, the aorta, crura of the diaphragm.

   Posterior to stomach, pancreas (upper border), left renal vein.

   The plexus surrounds the coeliac artery and the superior mesenteric artery.
   b. A – Kidney
   B – Liver
   C – Gallbladder
   D – Aorta.
   The renal artery may be seen in front of the vertebral body and the pancreas more anterior.

c. There is a tumour where the right should be. This could be a pancreatic cyst, adrenal or kidney tumour.

3. It receives the (a) sympathetic preganglionic white rami, (b) parasympathetic nerves. It is formed from the union of
   - Greater splanchnic nerve (T 5–8th thoracic sympathetic ganglia).
   - Lesser splanchnic nerve (T 10–11th thoracic sympathetic ganglia).
   - Least splanchnic nerve (12th thoracic sympathetic ganglion).
   Coeliac branch of vagus nerve (parasympathetic).

4. ▪ Patient explanation and consent.
   - Cannulate a vein and fluid infusion in progress.
   - Equipment for resuscitation, image intensifier.
   - Position lying prone with the abdomen supported by one or more pillows to prevent lordosis of the lumber spine.
   - Landmarks.
   - Locate the spinous process of T12, which lies over (posterior to) the body of L1. Mark a point 8 cm lateral to the mid line, below the 12th rib. This will be below the level of T12. Clean the skin. A 15–20 cm needle entering at this point is angled at 45–50° to the coronal plane and passed cephalad to a projected point anterior to T12/L1.
   - The needle should miss the transverse process and strike the body of L1 or T12 beyond the waist. A second needle should be introduced in the other side so that the blocking fluid spreads evenly. This is important if cancer has inflated the space and limits the spread of fluid from one side.
   - Redirect the needle to slide off the body until it stops 1–2 cm anterior to the body of L1 on a lateral film. Loss of resistance to the injection of air will be detected as the needle enters the retroperitoneal space.
   - On an AP film the needle should lie within the vertebral body medial to the edge of the pedicle.
   - 0.5 ml radio-opaque material (Niopam) confirms the position of the needle in the retroperitoneal space as the fluid spreads up and down in a narrow band seen on the lateral film. Check the fluid does not disappear into the abdomen or into the circulation through a vessel.
   - Aspirate as aorta or vena cava can be pierced by the needle.
   - Inject 2–3 ml LA as a larger injection will make the patient feel as if they have been kicked in the stomach.
   - A temporary block is achieved with 20 ml LA or a permanent block with 20 ml 50% alcohol.
   - Monitor BP which will fall due to vaso-dilatation below the diaphragm.

5. ▪ Intravascular injection
   - Intraperitoneal injection
   - Retroperitonal haematoma
   - Back ache
   - Neuritis on L1 root
   - Impotence
   - Trauma to pancreas or kidney due to the needle or alcohol injection misplaced.

Answers – Anatomy 5

1. The stellate ganglion is made up of the inferior cervical ganglion and the first thoracic ganglion.

2. Posterior. Neck of first rib and transverse process of first thoracic vertebra.

   Importance. All sympathetic efferents to head, neck and arm pass through this ganglion.

3. Block produces arm vasodilatation, reduction in sympathetic pain.

   Head and neck vasodilatation.

   Horner's syndrome: meiosis, enophthalmos, ptosis and dryness of the skin of the cheek.

   Nasal stuffiness due to the vasodilatation.

4. Indications for block:
   - Arm pain due to ischaemia
   - Frostbite
   - Inappropriate intra-arterial injection
   - Complex regional pain syndrome
   - Headache
   - Angina by spread to ganglia at T2–4.

5. Consent and explanation. Precautions for resuscitation.

   Site of block.

   Stellate ganglion block is performed with the patient inclined to 45°.

   The level of the cricoid is marked, or two fingers lateral to the sternal notch and above the clavicle.

   Sternomastoid and the carotid sheath are taken laterally by the index and middle fingers.

   Clean area. A 20–22 g 10 cm needle is introduced at the level of the cricoid until it hits the transverse process of C6. Withdraw by 1–2 mm before injection. This is not the level of the stellate ganglion but it is safe as it is above the dome of the pleura. 5–10 ml of local anaesthetic infiltrated in the sitting position will run, under gravity, to the stellate ganglion.

   A needle can be introduced down to C7 if an image intensifier is used.

6. Problems: pneumothorax, intravascular injection, particularly carotid or vertebral artery.

Answers – Anatomy 6

1. *Descending – Motor tracts*
   A – Lateral corticospinal tract
   B – Anterior cortico spinal tract
   C – Tectospinal tract

   Ascending – Sensory tracts
   D – Fasciculus gracilis
   E – Fasciculus cuneatus
   F – Posterior spino-cerebellar tract
   G – Anterior spino-cerebellar tract
   H – Lateral spino-thalamic tract
   I – Anterior spino-thalamic tract

2. Spinal cord in adult human is approximately 45 cm long.

3. Origin – continuation of brain stem at the foramen magnum. The dura fuses with the cranium inside the skull so the foramen magnum is the highest point of the epidural space.

   End – at the level of L1–L2 in adults, (L5/S1 in babies) the cord forms the conus medullaris and at S2 the dura ends and forms the filum terminale.

4. In transverse section, the grey matter occupies a central H-shaped area.

   The grey matter is made up of Nerve cells.

   It is divided into:
   - 2 posterior horns carrying the posterior columns, sensory fibres from the posterior roots.
   - 2 anterior horns carrying the anterior columns, motor cells, which will leave in the ventral roots.
   - In the thoracic region there are 2 lateral horns carrying the sympathetic nerves.

5. The white matter is composed of medullated nerve cells in a longitudinal orientation. It is divided into three column regions: posterior, anterior and lateral.
   a. Posterior columns. Two ascending tracts – fasciculus gracilis (medial) and fasiculus cuneatus (lateral) run to the medulla, synapses cross to the thalamus, then to the sensory cortex.
      Transmit:
      - Fine touch
      - Proprioception
   b. Lateral columns. Ascending – lateral spinothalamic tract.
      Transmit :
      - Pain and temperature
   c. Anterior columns. Two ascending tracts. Anterior and posterior spino-cerebellar tracts.
      Transmit:
      - Proprioception from muscle and joint are crossing fibres.

Anterior spinothalamic tract
Transmits:
- Light touch and pressure

Descending tracts
- Pyramidal tract is the major motor pathway
  - **i.** Cortico-spinal tracts
    - Lateral corticospinal
    - Anterior corticospinal
  - **ii.** Reticulo-spinal tract
  - **iii.** Tecto-spinal tract
  - **iv.** Rubro-spinal tract
  - **v.** Vestibulo-spinal tract

Answers – Anatomy 7

1. **A** – Internal carotid artery
   B – Basilar artery
   C – Vertebral artery
   D – Anterior spinal artery
   E – Anterior communicating artery
   F – Posterior communicating artery
   G – Posterior cerebral artery
   H – Superior cerebellar artery
   I – Pontine arteries
   J – Anterior inferior cerebellar artery
   K – posterior inferior cerebellar artery.

2. The circle of Willis is supplied by arterial blood from:
   - Two internal carotid arteries
   - Two vertebral arteries leading to the basilar artery
   - The pressure and flow of blood on each side is equalised by the circle of Willis. But if one carotid artery is acutely blocked the flow in the other is not sufficient to prevent hemiplegia.

3. The carotid artery enters the cranium through the carotid foramen and divides into three branches: anterior and middle cerebral and posterior communicating arteries. Other branches enter the brain to the internal capsule and caudate nucleus.

   The vertebral arteries enter the cranium through the foramen magnum. They join to form the basilar artery. Each vertebral artery gives an anterior spinal artery and a posterior inferior cerebellar artery.

   The Basilar artery branches:
   - Posterior cerebral
   - Superior cerebellar
   - Anterior internal cerebellar
   - Labyrinthine
   - Pontine arteries.

   Blood supply to the spinal cord.

4. **A** – Posterior spinal artery
   B – Posterior spinal vein
   C – Anterior spinal vein
   D – Anterior spinal artery
   E – Area supplied by the anterior spinal artery. The anterior spinal artery supplies blood to two-thirds of the cord.

   Blood supply
   The spinal cord receives arterial supply from:
   - Anterior spinal arteries
   - Posterior spinal arteries

with an additional contribution from spinal branches of:

- Vertebral arteries
- Intercostal arteries
- Lumbar arteries
- Sacral arteries
- Radicular arteries. Serve to reinforce the anterior spinal artery supply at the low thoracic and high lumbar level. One of these is large – the arteria radicularis magna – and supplies two-thirds of the cord.

Venous drainage

Complex anterior and posterior spinal veins drain to

- Segmental veins which drain to
  - Azygous veins
  - Lumbar veins
  - Sacral veins.

5. Causes uncertain:
   - Thrombosis of anterior spinal artery
   - Spasm of anterior spinal artery
   - Effect of hypotension
   - Vasoconstrictor drugs given systemically
   - LA with epinephrine.

Symptoms and signs

- Lower limb paresis
- Variable sensory deficit
- Noticeable as the normal blockage resolves.

6. Complete loss of all sensory and voluntary movement below the level of the lesion
   - State of spinal shock which lasts up to 4 weeks
   - Flaccidity of muscles
   - Absent reflexes
   - Autonomic dysfunction
     - Hypotension
     - Bradycardia
     - Hypothermia
     - Bladder retention
     - Paralytic ileus
   - Oedema.

Recovery phase

- Spastic
- Autonomic hyper-reflexia
- Increased BP
- Increased HR
- Increased sweating.

Hemisection

Neurological deficit on different sides depending on whether the nerve pathways cross in the cord.

Deficit on the same side as the lesion affects the pathways that do not cross:

- Pyramidal tracts – ipsilateral paralysis
- Posterior columns loss of proprioception and fine discrimination – ipsilateral sensory loss.

Deficit on the other side to the lesion with pathways that cross.

Spinothalmic tract with loss of pain and temperature – contralateral sensory loss.

7. CSF:
   - Total volume 180–200 ml
     - Brain – 100 ml
     - Vertebral canal – 35 ml
   - Production   500 ml/day
                   30 ml/h

   pH 7.31
   SG 1006
   - CSF > Cl^-, Mg^{+2} and urea than plasma.
   CSF < protein 0.2–0.4 g/l than plasma.
   CSF <glucose 2.2–4.4 mmol/l than plasma.

Answers – Anatomy 8

1. **A** – Right coronary artery
   B – Left circumflex artery
   C – Left anterior descending or intervertebral artery
   D – Marginal branch of right coronary artery.
   E – Left main stem, coronary artery.

2. An inferior myocardial infarction. The majority of people will get AV node and Bundle of Hiss conduction disturbances due to right coronary artery dominance.

3. ECG. ST elevation in II, III and a VF. Stages of heart block from long PR interval to compete heart block. RBBB.

4. An anterior infarction. ECG changes in the anterior standard chest leads V2 to V5.

5. The Thesbian circulation is that part of the coronary venous circulation that drains directly into the cardiac chambers.

6. One or two per cent of cardiac output.

7. The blood draining into the left-sided chambers represents an anatomical shunt.

8. The bronchial circulation.

9. Parasympathetic, cardiac inhibitor, from the vagus nerve. Sympathetic from the upper thoracic ganglia 2, 3 and 4 which supply a superficial and deep cardiac plexus.

10. The ejection fraction is the stroke volume – normally 70 ml divided by the left ventricular volume – normally 100 ml. This gives a normal of 70%.

11. Ejection fraction is determined by echocardiography.

12. This is a left coronary arteriogram from a left anterior oblique projection. The main stem (1) divides into: left anterior descending (3) and circumflex (2).

13. The left coronary artery arises from the left posterior aortic sinus. It passes lateral to the pulmonary trunk and runs in the left atrioventricular groove.

    The main stem divides in two arteries. The left anterior descending artery which supplies the anterior wall of the left ventricle and the interventricular septum. The circumflex artery which supplies the later wall of the left ventricle.

    The right coronary artery arises from the anterior aortic sinus. It passes between the pulmonary trunk and the right atrium. Then in the right atrioventricular grove between the right atrium and the ventricle. It descends on the anterior surface of the heart and continues along the inferior border to anastomose with the left coronary artery.

It supplies the right ventricle, the SA node, the AV node, the posterior and inferior parts of the left ventricle.

The aortic sinuses are above the attached margins of the cusps of the aortic valve.

14. The sinuatrial node (horse-shoe shaped) is in the upper part of the crista terminalis (sulcus terminalis) of the right atrium extending medially around the opening of the SVC. It extends through the thickness of atrial wall from epicardium to endocardium.

15. The atrioventricular node lies above the orifice of the coronary sinus in the fibres of the artrial septum. From the node the AV bundle passes to the membranous part of the interventricular septum where it divides. The right and left limbs (fasiculi) run into the right and left ventricles on each side of the septum. The right limb passes in the moderator band to the base of the anterior papillary muscle. The left limb passes to the apex of the ventricle. The terminal fibres are the Purkinje fibres, which spread out beneath the endocardium.

16. The right coronary artery supplies the SA, AV bodies, the AV bundle and the right branch. The left bundle is supplied by both coronary arteries.

17. Layers of the heart are the epicardium – fibrous pericardium with a thin serous layer, myocardium – muscle fibres, endocardium – a thin endothelium covering connective and elastic fibres.

18. The mitral valve has two main triangular cusps, a large anterior and a smaller posterior cusp. Two smaller cusps are found in the angles between the larger cusps. Chordae tendinae are attached to the cusps and through papillary muscles to the ventricle wall. They prevent the cusps passing into the atrium.

    The aortic valve has three semilunar cusps, two posterior and one anterior. The tricuspid valve has three cusps and the pulmonary valve three cusps.

    Sinuses of Valsalva are dilatations at the beginning of the aorta and pulmonary artery, behind each valve cusp. The three aortic sinuses are bigger than the three pulmonary sinuses. Blood is pushed back into the sinuses during diastole. This assists the closing of the valve flaps to prevent regurgitation.

19. The septomarginal trabecula or moderator band is a muscular band running from the inter-ventricular septum to the base of the anterior papillary muscle in the right ventricle. This muscle band may prevent over-filling of the ventricle. The band also carries the right branch after the atrioventricular bundle has divided into left and right. The bundle can be excited and lead to ectopic beats by the touch of an intracardiac catheter.

20. Venous drainage.

    About two-thirds of the venous drainage of the heart is by veins, which accompany the coronary arteries. These veins drain into the coronary sinus, which lies in the posterior AV groove. The sinus drains into the right atrium through an opening between the inferior vena cava and the atrioventricular opening. The opening is covered by a semicircular valve, which prevents regurgitation of blood during atrial contraction. The coronary sinus drains the great cardiac vein, the middle cardiac vein, the small cardiac vein and the oblique cardiac vein.

The anterior cardiac vein drains directly into the right atrium.

The rest of the blood drains by small veins into the cardiac cavities.

21. Normally venous blood is 75% saturated. It is much lower in the coronary sinus where the saturation can be as low as 40% depending on myocardial work.

Answers – Anatomy 9

1. The brachial plexus.

2. C5 to C8 and T1.

3. *A.* Ulnar
   B. Radial
   C. Musculocutaneous
   D. Lateral cord
   E. Medial cutaneous nerve of the forearm
   F. Median nerve
   G. Medial cutaneous nerve of the arm.

4. The nerve roots emerge from the neck through the intervertebral foramina, which lie between the transverse processes in the neck. The nerve roots lie posterior to the vertebral artery, then between scalenus anterior and scalenus medius. In the neck the plexus lies above the subclavian artery.

At the clavicle the plexus lies anterior to scalenus medius with the subclavian artery anteriorly. Medially is the pleura.

In the axilla the cords surround the axillary artery which lies deep to the axillary vein.

The lateral and posterior cords lie lateral to the axillary artery and the medial cord lies behind the artery. Laterally and anteriorly is coracobrachialis and posteriorly is teres minor.

5. *a.* Posterior triangle, posterior to sternomastoid. Transverse processes, particularly C6 at the level of the cricoid cartilage.
   b. Posterior to the subclavian artery as it passes over the clavicle. Or extend the external jugular vein to give the mid point of the clavicle.
   c. Palpate the axillary artery as high as possible in the axilla between corachobrachialis and teres minor.

6. Intercostobrachial nerve supplying the superior and medial surface of the arm, musculocutaneous nerve supplying the radial side of the forearm.

7. Ulnar and median nerves.

8. Consent and explanation, resuscitation equipment. Patient supine, pillow under head.

Arm abducted to 90°.

Elbow flexed, shoulder rotated to allow the dorsum of the hand to rest on the pillow.

Palpate the axillary artery in the axillary groove as high as possible in the axilla between latissimus dorsi with teres major underneath forming the posterior axillary fold and pectoralis major forming the anterior axillary fold.

Inject a 23 gauge needle alongside the artery. Feel a give, a click and test for loss of resistance to injection. Inject 20 ml LA keeping a finger distal to the injection to encourage the LA to flow proximally. A catheter can be used for repeated injection.

Problems with the axillary block
Miss the circumflex, radial and muscular cutaneous nerve of forearm, leaves sensation on radial side of forearm.

Miss intercostal brachial nerve, sensation on superior and medial arm.

Complications haematoma and intravascular injection, failure due to injection outside the sheath.

9. Consent and explanation, resuscitation equipment.

   Patient supine, head tilted facing slightly away from the side to be blocked, shoulder depressed.

   Palpate the cricoid cartilage and draw a line posterior to join with the posterior border of Sternomastoid.

   The interscalene groove if felt slightly dorsal, medial and caudal.

   A 23 g needle is injected medial and caudal (to avoid entering the vertebral artery), towards the transverse process of C6 in this groove, at the level of the cricoid.

   Aspirate to avoid injecting into vertebral artery or CSF. Nerve stimulator will cause contraction of biceps, triceps or deltoid.

10. Problems: failure to block C8/T1 the hand and superior/medial upper arm.

Complications
- Epidural, spinal, intravascular – vertebral artery injection
- Phrenic nerve block
- Recurrent laryngeal nerve
- Horner's syndrome
- Pneumothorax.

11. Identify the mid point of the clavicle by marking the distal end of the clavicle and the sternal notch, palpation of the subclavian artery passing over the first rib or extrapolation forward of the external jugular vein.

    The brachial plexus passes over the first rib behind the subclavian artery, which in turn is behind the vein.

    The patient lies supine with the head towards the opposite side. IV access, equipment for resuscitation. Clean the area. 1 cm above the mid point of the clavicle, with a finger on the artery, introduce a fine gauge needle vertically downwards towards the first rib. Do not point inwards as here lies the pleura. Once the rib is identified move the needle anterior or posterior with a nerve stimulator until the plexus is identified by hand movement. A fine gauge needle will often allow the feeling of a click as the sheath is entered.

How is this different from the subclavian, perivascular block?
The subclavian perivascular block uses the subclavian artery behind the clavicle and the interscalene groove as landmarks. The needle is introduced more posterio-medially than for the subclavian approach. It is passed caudally between the scalene muscles and behind the artery. If the needle is in the interscalene groove it should be felt to enter the sheath with a "give" and paraesthesiae obtained before reaching the first rib. A successful position is indicated by the hands twitching to a stimulus of the middle trunk.

Indications: Upper and lower arm and hand. The lower trunk may be missed and so the ulnar leaving little finger sensation.

Problems pneumothorax, intravascular injection and haematomas.

12. As for any LA block, IV injection and CNS, CVS effects. Pneumothorax, stellate ganglion block and Horner's syndrome, phrenic nerve block. Back-tracking of LA to the epidural space. Intravascular injection.

13. A safe dose of local anaesthetic assumes that it is not injected into a vessel. Doses for LA infiltrated into the tissues.

Lidocaine 3 mg/kg without epinephrine and 6 mg/kg with epinephrine. Bupivacaine 2 mg/kg/4 h.

Prilocaine is said to be safer than lidocaine but can produce methaemoglobinaemia 6 mg/kg plain and 9 mg/kg with epinephrine.

Procaine may be safer as it is metabolised by pseudocholinesterase when it enters the circulation.

Epinephrine should not be added around end arteries or injected into the epidural space or intrathecal spaces due to the unpredictable arterial supply to the spinal cord.

Adding epinephrine to bupivacaine in the epidural space is unnecessary, as the duration of action of bupivacaine is longer than epinephrine.

Answers – Anatomy 10

1. T12 to S4.

2. L1 to L4 form the lumbar plexus. This gives rise to the femoral nerve and obturator nerve L2, 3, 4.

L4 to S4 form the sacral plexus. This gives rise to the sciatic nerve L4, 5 and S2, 3, 4 and pudendal nerve S 2, 3, 4.

Other nerves:
- Ilio-inguinal and ilio-hypogastric nerves L1 supply skin of the upper and medial thigh.
- Lateral cutaneous nerve of thigh L2, 3 supplies the skin of the lateral thigh.

Femoral nerve. Three components: motor, sensory and articular.

Passes through psoas muscle and under the inguinal ligament.

Motor: anterior compartment of thigh: quadriceps, sartorius, pectineus.

Sensory: Medial and intermediate cutaneous nerves of the thigh, saphenous nerve.

Articular to the knee and ankle joints.

Obturator nerve passes from the medial edge of psoas around the lateral wall of the pelvis to the obturator foramen.

Motor: Adductor longus, gracilis, adductor brevis and adductor magnus.

Articular: Hip and knee joint.

Sciatic nerve descends over the pelvic brim towards the greater sciatic notch.

Mid-thigh it divides into the tibial nerve and the common peroneal nerve.

Motor to piriformis, gluteal muscles, biceps femoris, semitendinosus, semimembranosus.

Sensory to perineum and posterior leg.

In the popliteal fossa superficial to the popliteal artery and vein.

Motor to gastrocnemius, soleus.

Sensory: Sural nerve past lateral malleolus to 5th toe.

Articular to knee.

Medial and lateral plantar nerves posterior to medial malleolus behind tibial artery.

Sensory to heel, medial sole and part of lateral sole.

Deep peroneal nerve from common peroneal nerve. Passes over ankle behind flexor hallucis longus, supplies the medial half of the dorsum of the foot and the 1st and 2nd digits.

Superficial peroneal nerve branch of common peroneal nerve.

Pudendal nerve supplies the perineum.

Answers – Anatomy 11

1. **A** – Biceps muscle
   B – Cephalic vein
   C – Brachioradialis
   D – Median nerve
   E – Basilic vein
   F – Brachial artery
   G – Pronator teres – humeral head overlying the medial epicondyle and the common tendon of the forearm flexors
   H – Pronator teres.

   Note that medial to the biceps tendon from lateral to medial: artery, nerve, vein.

   Pronator teres and brachio radialis muscles border the antecubital fossa.

2. **A** – Median nerve
   B – Radial nerve
   C – Ulnar nerve.

3. The upper limb is drained by groups of:
   - Superficial veins
   - Deep veins

   These systems eventually meet as the axillary vein which becomes the subclavian vein at the lateral border of the first rib.
   a. Superficial group of veins.
   The precise arrangement of these veins is variable but usually as follows:
   - Blood drains from the fingers through digital veins, which lie superficially on the back of the hand
   - These join to form the dorsal venous arch
   - From which arises the cephalic vein and basilic vein.

4. Superficial veins

Cephalic vein	Basilic vein
Travels up the radial side of forearm	Travels up the ulnar side of forearm
Passes anterior to antecubital fossa	Passes anterior to antecubital fossa
Lies lateral to biceps muscle in upper arm	Lies medial to biceps muscle in upper arm
Travels medially in delto-pectoral groove	May be crossed by anterior and posterior branches of medial cutaneous nerve of forearm at the elbow
Pierces clavipectoral fascia and joins axillary vein	In mid upper arm pierces deep fascia to join brachial veins forming the axillary vein

Overlying the antecubital fossa.

The cephalic and basilic veins communicate by means of:

- Median cubital vein. It receives tributaries from the forearm as well as a deep vein.
- Median basilic vein. It runs proximally and medially to join the basilic vein.
- Median cephalic vein. It usually arises from the cephalic vein distal to the epicondyl (lateral).

5. - Radial and ulnar veins run up the forearm alongside their corresponding arteries. They join at the elbow to form the brachial vein.
   - Brachial vein receives the basilic vein and continues as axillary vein from the lower border of teres major.

6. Radial nerve
   - Runs first between axillary artery and axillary vein
   - Then on medial aspect of brachial artery as far as the insertion of coracobrachialis into the humerus at the mid point of the humerus
   - Then passes backwards to pierce the medial intermuscular septum
   - Lies on the anterior face of the medial head of triceps
   - Behind the medial epicondyl of the humerus
   - Between the humoral and ulnar heads at flexor carpi ulnaris
   - To supply flexor digitorum profundum.

7. The brachial artery is the continuation of axillary artery.

   May bifurcate high in the arm even at axillary level into two:
   - Main trunk
     - Continues in the forearm as the Common Interosseous Artery
   - Common stem
     - Superficial brachial artery

   Ends at the neck of the radius or upper arm by dividing into the radial and ulnar arteries.

   It is superficial (immediately below the deep fascia) along the whole of its course except where crossed by the median nerve at the mid-humerus which passes superiorly from lateral to medial. Just above the antecubital fossa, along the medial border of biceps the order from lateral to medial is brachial artery, median nerve, and basilic vein.

Answers – Anatomy 12

1. **A** – Flexor carpi radialis tendon
   B – Radial artery
   C – Flexor carpi ulnaris tendon
   D – Ulnar artery
   E – Palmaris longus
   F – Median nerve.

2. The ulnar nerve overlies the ulnar artery and flexor carpi ulnaris. Abductor pollucis is lateral to the radial artery.

STATISTICS

11

Statistics 1

(Answers on page 339)

Questions

1. What preparation is required before starting a trial?

2. What criteria should be used for inclusion and exclusion in a drug trial?

3. What is randomisation and how can it be achieved?

4. What are the phases of clinical trials?

5. What are the characteristics of the two types of statistics?

6. What are the mean, mode and median and how are they defined?

7. What are measures of dispersion (variation or spread)?

8. What are normal distribution characteristics and skewed distribution characteristics?

9. What errors can occur in sampling?

10. What are the null hypothesis and the types of error that may occur?

11. What does a P value of 0.05 mean?

12. What tests can be used to test for significance of parametric data?

13. Describe the method for using a Chi-squared test.

14. Draw a plot of Y against X for a high positive and a high negative correlation.

Answers
Statistics

Answers – Statistics 1

1. Background and general aims. Why is the trial needed? How does it build on previous knowledge? Literature search to ascertain the present state of knowledge.

   Specific objectives. Exact description of the hypotheses that are being tested. It is always statistically more significant to answer specific questions rather than globally trawl for data and then fit questions to the results.

   Protocol for ethical approval must include a patient explanation and consent form and details of funding.

2. Criteria for patient selection
   a. What kind of people are to be sampled? The sample population must be representative of:
      i.   Patients likely to benefit from the therapy being trialled.
      ii. A carefully defined disease state.
   b. Consent with a written explanation. All the patients selected must be suitable for the treatment(s).
   c. Age group, sex.
   d. Exclude factors that could bias the results of the trial, e.g. other diseases or drug therapies. Patients who could be harmed by the treatment, e.g. pregnancy.

   Treatment schedules
   a. An exact plan of how the treatments will be given and an escape therapy.

   Evaluation of response
   a. A plan of:-
      i.   What will be measured, both as a baseline and after treatment?
      ii. How will it be measured? Has the method been validated?
      iii. Who will do the measuring to ensure lack of bias?
   b. The evaluation should be divided measuring the:
      iv. Principle response
      v.   Side-effects
   c. What methods are to be used to ensure accuracy and reduce the risk of bias?

   Trial design and how treatment will be allocated to prevent bias.
   ▪ Blinding – Open, blind, double blind, cross-over, cohort and descriptive.
   ▪ Use of control groups. What will they have? Is a placebo ethical?

- ■ Method of randomisation.
- ■ Required size of study. Assess the estimated number of subjects from the P value (α-error) and the power (β-error).

Form for data entry. Should be designed and assessed to remove any ambiguity.

- ■ Protocol deviations. What to do with those patients that do not follow the planned regime? **Intention to treat** means once a patient has been allocated a place it cannot be used by another patient.

Plans for statistical analysis. To ensure that the questions asked are those that are answered, not those that happen to be thrown up by the results.

Administrative responsibility.

Funding and financial incentives.

3. Randomisation is the process by which the subjects in a drug trial are allocated to receive either:
- ■ The study drug
- ■ The control.

The allocation should be by chance to minimise bias.

In a matched pair design there is no randomisation.

<u>Open trial</u>: everyone knows what is being used.

<u>Single blind study</u>: the subject does not know whether they receive a trial or a control agent.

<u>Double blind study</u>: neither the subject nor the observer knows the nature of the drug administered.

4. *Phase I*
Aim to work out the pharmacokinetics, pharmacodynamics, tolerance and safety.
Subjects – Healthy volunteers and or fit patients.
Number – 50–100.
Investigator – Research scientist such as a clinical pharmacologist.

The acute effects of the agent are studied over a broad range of doses. Starting with a dose that produces no effect and increasing to produce either a major therapeutic response or a very minor toxic effect.

Phase II
Aim to describe the efficacy, dose–response relationship and safety.
Subjects – Patients who may benefit.
Number < 200.
Investigator – Research scientist such as a clinical pharmacologist.

In phase II a placebo or control drug is used in a single or double blind study. The aim is to determine if the agent has an effect at doses acceptable to the sick patient.

Phase III
Aim to determine the efficacy and safety on a larger population.
Subjects – patients.
Numbers – 2000–5000.
Investigators – Clinicians in the specialty.

These studies usually include a placebo or positive controls in a double-blind cross-over design. The goal is to explore the spectrum of beneficial action of the new drug and compare it with established therapies.

Phase IV
Aim to collect information on the use of the drug in clinical practice.
Subjects – Patients.
Number – >2000.
Investigators – Clinicians in the field.

It is hoped that infrequent events will be detected.

5. *Types of statistics*

Descriptive statistics	Inferential statistics
Describes and presents the data Tables, diagrams, numbers	Draws conclusions from the data
Central tendency and dispersion distributions	Variables and parameters Parametric and non parametric
Identifies the presence or otherwise of a central tendency in data and generates mean, median and mode	Makes deductions from a sample about a population SEM Confidence limits

A population is a group of subjects.

Variable is a quantity, which varies, e.g. BP or pulse.

Parameter is a measurement or an outcome, which summarises or characterises the population, e.g. mean BP or correlation of BP with age.

Examples of types of data

Qualitative (Categorical)		Quantitative (Discrete or continuous)	
Nominal Mutually exclusive variables Non-parametric	**Ordinal** ranking scale. Variable: higher than, better than	**Parametric** Interval or Continuous	**Non-parametric** Cannot add or take a mean
Sex (male/female)	None, mild, moderate, severe	Continuous Blood pressure	Number of patients who vomit
Marital status	Better/worse	Height	Number of children with asthma

Qualitative (Categorical)		Quantitative (Discrete or continuous)
Blood group	Agree/neutral, disagree	Weight
Response Yes/No Alive/dead		Interval Age group
Nausea or headache: Subjective, Nominal categorical: no agreed order of severity	Pain score: Ordinal, subjective	

Presentation

Qualitative (Nominal, Categorical) Data

Bar and pie charts or histogram.

Histogram. The height of each block is proportional to the frequency of the score.

Shows the distribution of a discrete variable.

Cumulative frequency is plotted for each step
- The frequency of data at each step represents the sum of that step added to previous steps.
- These data are used to produce percentile charts using the median results.

Scales
- Arithmetic
  - Equal distances measure equal absolute distances.
- Logarithmic usually to base 10
  - Equal distance measures equal proportional differences (percentage change in the variable). Tends to straighten an exponential or skewed curve.
- Presentation
  - Parametric Interval Scale Data can be presented as mean, mode, and median.

6. Measures of central tendency
Central tendency describes the typical value from the data group. It may be calculated as:
- **Mean** is the "average" of a population.

$$\text{Arithmetic mean} = \frac{\text{Sum of observations}}{\text{Number of observations}}$$

- **Median** lies exactly halfway when the values are ranked in order.
  - It gives no measure of the extreme values in a series of results.
  - In any symmetrical distribution the mean, median and mode will be the same.

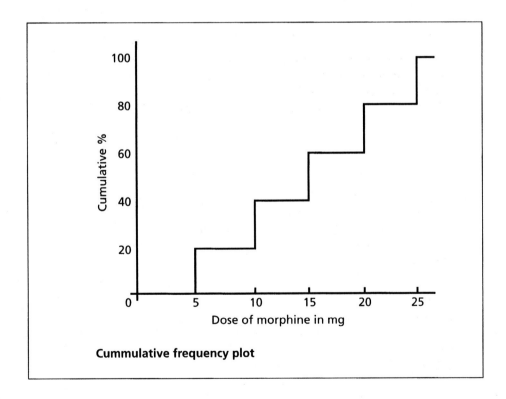

Histogram

Cummulative frequency plot

- The mean–median difference is a rather crude measurement of the "skewness" of the population.
- **Mode** is the most commonly observed measurement in a series of values. It is not particularly useful. It is the peak on a frequency distribution curve. But there may be two peaks – bimodal, or many peaks – multimodal.

7. Measures of the dispersion of the data about the central tendency.
   - Sample range
   - Percentile
   - Variance and standard deviation
   - Coefficient of variation.
   a. Sample range is the difference between the highest and lowest values. Disadvantages
      - Range will increase as the size of the population increases
      - It provides no information as to the values between the extremes.
   b. Percentile is the percentage of results that lie below that level.
      - A quartile is the percentage of results at 25%, 50%, and 75%.
      - The "interquartile range" contains 50% of the observations between 25% and 75%.
      - Relationship between mean, median, and mode.
         - Symmetrical distribution. Mean = mode = median
         - Moderately skewed distribution. Mean – mode = 3 (mean – median).
   c. Variance and standard deviation are measures of the sampling error by assessing the spread of the observations about the mean.
      - Variance σ^2
         i. A measure of the variation about the mean
         ii. Derived by squaring all the deviations from the mean, adding the results and dividing by the number of results.

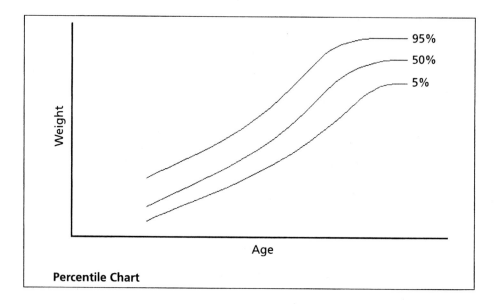

Percentile Chart

iii. $\dfrac{\text{Sum of (Individual observation – Mean)}^2}{\text{Number of observation}} = \dfrac{\text{Sum } (x - \bar{x})^2}{\text{Number}}$

S = is the estimate of population variance based on sample statistics.

iv. Standard deviation (SD or σ) is a measure of the spread of the values around the mean. It is the square root of the variance.

d. Coefficient of variation is the SD divided by the mean of the observations expressed as

a percentage $= \dfrac{\text{SD}}{\text{Mean}} \times 100\%$

- Expressed as a percentage.
- Used to make comparisons of spread when the means are dissimilar, i.e. SD of 5 around a mean of 50 indicates a greater degree of scatter than SD of 5 around a mean of 500.

8. Normal or Gaussian distribution

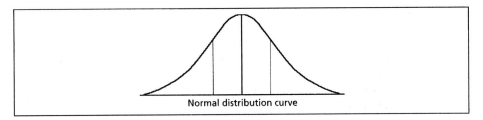

Normal distribution curve

- The curve has a convex top and concave tail.
- This is theoretically a symmetrical, bell-shaped distribution.
- The normal distribution curve is symmetrical around the mean.
- Specified by its mean and standard deviation. Mean, median and mode are equal.

Approximately

- 68% of the observation fall within one SD of the mean
- 95% of the observation fall within two SD from the mean
- 99.7% of the observation fall within three SD from the mean.

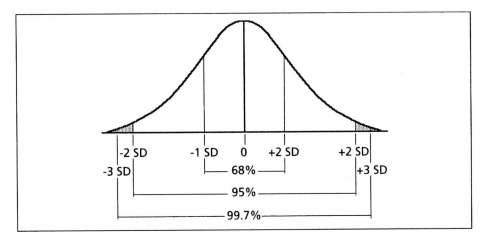

Skewed distribution is a distribution that is asymmetrical.

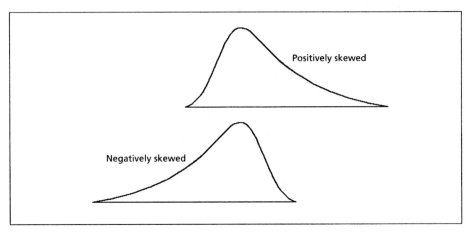

- A **negatively** skewed distribution has a longer tail among the **lower** values.
- A **positively** skewed distribution has a longer tail among the **higher** values.
- In a skewed curve
  - The mean is always towards the long tail
  - The mode nearer the short tail
  - The median is between the two.

Log-Normal distribution
- This is a skewed distribution when plotted using an arithmetic scale
- BUT it is a normal distribution using a logarithmic scale to eliminate skewing.

Binomial distribution applies when there are only two outcomes to a trial e.g. cure or death.

Poisson distribution
- The probability of occurrence of a **rare event** in a large population.

9. Sampling is used to estimate the occurrence of an event.

Statistical inference is the process of inferring characteristics of a population by the observation of a sample.

Sampling errors may be due to
- Systematic errors (biases)
- Random errors.

Systematic errors (biases)
a. Selection bias occurs when comparisons are made between groups of patients who have a difference other than the one studied.

  Methods for reducing selection bias:
  - Randomisation.
  - Limit the type of patient studied – many exclusions.

- Match patients in one group with those in a comparison group.
- Stratification involves comparing rates within groups of individuals who have the same values for the main variable.
- Adjustment. Using simple methods of standardisation, or techniques of multiple linear and logistic regression.

b. Measurement bias occurs when the methods of measurement are consistently dissimilar among groups of patients. Could occur with recording pain scores if a measuring scale has not been validated.

c. Confounding bias occurs when two factors occur together and the effect of one is confused or distorted by the other.

Random errors are determined by
- Heterogeneity of the population.
- Sample size.

Standard error of the mean (SEM)
- Defined as standard deviation divided by square root of the number of observation

$$SEM = \frac{SD}{\sqrt{\text{sample size } n}}$$

More correctly – Standard deviation divided by the $\sqrt{}$ degrees of freedom or *n*-1.
- The confidence that the mean of the sample reflects the mean of the whole population. Or how accurate is the sample mean as an estimate of the population mean?
- The SD is a measure of the **variability** of the observations.
- The distribution of the means of samples has a SD around the population mean, which describes the distribution of mean values.
- It is also used when one sample mean is compared to another and in constructing a confidence interval for a mean or proportion.
- The SE of the mean of one sample is an estimate of the SD that would be obtained from the means of a large number of samples drawn from the population.

Factors affecting SEM
i. Sample size (*n*). As *n* increases, SEM decreases.
ii. SD of the original population values. As the SD increases, the SEM increases.

Hypothesis testing and statistical significance.

10. Null hypothesis
- States that "there is no difference between the samples or populations being compared and that any difference observed is simply the result of random variation".

P1 is the probability of the characteristic in a sample or population.

P2 is the probability of the same characteristic in the control sample or comparison population.

Null hypothesis (H_o) $P1 - P2 = 0$ or $P1 = P2$

Analytic statistical methods set out to disprove the Null hypothesis by demonstrating a difference.

Statistical significance
A test of significance is a method for deciding whether a difference exists between two groups. If there is a difference what is the probability that it happened by chance?

Type I error
* Difference exists when there is no difference.
* The probability of detecting a significant difference when the parameters or treatments are really the same.
* A false-positive result.
* Reject the null hypothesis when it is in fact true.

Significance level (α)
* Conventional significance levels are
  * 5%, P value 0.05.
  * 1%, P value 0.01.
  * 0.1%, P value 0.001.

The smaller the value the less the likelihood of the difference having occurred by chance.

A 5% significance level (P value 0.05):
* Most often used for statistical comparisons in medicine.
* There is a 5% chance of detecting a difference and rejecting the null hypothesis when the treatments are actually the same.

Means that:
* 1 out of 20 times the difference would occur by chance OR
* If the test were repeated 20 times it would produce a significant result once by chance alone.
* Chosen at the start of a study it is the risk of a type 1 error.

The commonest cause of type I error is *multiple testing or making too many readings until one set proves to be different.*

11. Critical value = Statistical probability (P value)
    * This is the number of 1 or less or a ratio, indicating the likelihood that a result should be expected. 1 means the result should be expected.
    * It is expressed as "P".
    * Can only be derived by inferential statistical methods.
    * It represents the ratio of the number of actual occurrences to the number of possible occurrences.
    * Conventional P values are 0.05 (5%), 0.01 (1%), 0.001 (0.1%).
    * The probability outcome in a statistical test of $P < 0.05$ is usually taken as significant. This means accepting as significant any result that occurs less frequently than once in 20 times.

- The level of probability determines the frequency with which the following errors occur:
  - type I (α)
  - type II (β).
- Critical region (rejection region) is a set of values of the test leading to rejection of the null hypothesis.

Type II error

- The probability of **not detecting** a significant difference when a difference really exists.
- The risk of a false negative result.

Cause: Insufficient sample size.

Avoided by performing a power analysis and including a large enough sample.

The power of the test is:

- the power of the test to detect a difference if it exists = (1 – type II error).
- power analysis should be performed *prior to starting clinical trial* to determine the numbers required in the study groups to show a specified difference (which is selected on the basis of the required clinically significant difference).
  It may also be applied retrospectively when assessing the validity of a statistically insignificant result.

The power of a test depends on the significance level, the size of the difference to be detected and the sample size.

An insufficient number of patients may lead to failure to detect a true difference that exists or type II error.
A clinically important result will usually mean a big difference. This is not necessarily the same as a statistically significant result.

One and two-tailed tests

a. A two-tailed test:
- Analyses the upper and lower results in the normal distribution to decide which of two treatments is best.

b. A one-tailed test:
- Analyses only one side of the normal distribution to decide if one treatment is better than placebo.
- The P value for a one sided test is generally **half** that for a two-sided test.

Confidence interval

- The interval or range about the sample mean, which contains the unknown true value, with a calculated probability.
- The range of values derived from sample data relating the data to the actual population.

Importance:
- It indicates the likely magnitude of differences between sample values by giving a range within which the true value lies.

Clinically used confidence limits are 90%, 95% and 99%.
- Sample mean ± 1.00 SE = 68% confidence interval (probability 0.68).
- Sample mean ± 1.96 SE = 95% confidence interval (probability 0.95). This is the commonest used level. That is 95% of sample means are within the normal distribution curve i.e. within a distance of ± 1.95 SE from the reference mean.
  or There is a 95% confidence that the interval contains the true (population) mean with a probability (P value) of 0.05.
- Sample mean ± 2.56 SE = 99% confidence interval (probability 0.99).

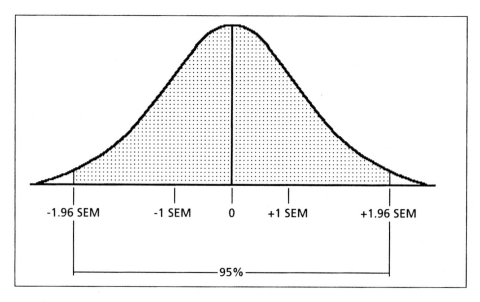

If a result occurs which has a value outside the 95% confidence limits it is in the 5% minority of the results. Or the probability of finding a result outside the 95% confidence limits is 5% which is written P < 0.05. The result is then significant at the 5% level.
- A confidence interval that is narrow emphasises the significance of the result.
- The P value describes the significance, not the confidence intervals around it.
- Confidence intervals are large if the sample size is small.

12. Analytical tests
- These are tests of inferential statistics (as opposed to descriptive statistics) designed to draw conclusions regarding differences between two or more sets of data.
- Used for making comparisons between sample means.
  Two types of data, two types of tests:
- **Parametric** – numerical characteristics of a given population.

■ **Non-parametric** – frequencies or scores which have no fixed numerical value.

Parametric tests are used when the following basic requirements are met:
a. The populations from which the samples are taken should be normally distributed.
b. The data are of the:
   i. Interval type
   ii. Continuous type
   iii. Ratio type
c. The variances of the samples are the same.
   ■ Student's t-test when two groups of data are involved.
   ■ Analysis of variance (ANOVA) when there are more than two groups of data.

Student's t-test
■ M Gossett (1908), a Guinness sampler in Dublin who signed himself "student" or "t" for short, devised the test.
■ It is the most sensitive test for detecting a genuine difference.
■ It is based on the t-distribution.
■ It is used for comparing a single small sample (< 60) with a large population.
■ To compare the difference in means between two small samples.
■ It cannot be used to compare more than two means.
■ As the sample size increases then the t distribution closely resembles the normal distribution.
■ At infinite degrees of freedom the t value and normal distribution are identical.

$$\text{calculated } t \text{ value} = \frac{\text{observed difference in means}}{\text{standard error of the difference in means}} \quad \frac{\bar{x}_1 - \bar{x}_2}{\sqrt{\dfrac{SD^2}{n_1}} + \sqrt{\dfrac{SD^2}{n_2}}}$$

■ The P value is obtained by using a table to match the calculated t value with the number of degrees of freedom.
■ The larger the value of t, and the smaller the value of P, the more likely there is a real difference.

Paired data
■ The paired t-test compares the means of two linked observations
   ● On the same individual
   ● On matched individuals.
It is more powerful than the standard 't' test. It might involve the same patient taking drug A and then drug B

$$t = \frac{\bar{x}}{\sqrt{\dfrac{S^2}{n}}}$$

$\bar{x}$ = the mean difference between the pairs.
S = SD.
n = the number of pairs.

Un-paired data

The unpaired t test compares the means of two separate groups of patients.

$$t = \frac{\bar{x}_1 - \bar{x}_2}{S\sqrt{\left(\dfrac{1}{n_1} + \dfrac{1}{n_2}\right)}}$$

S = the pooled SD.
n_1 and n_2 are the numbers of patients in each group.
$\bar{x}_1$ and $\bar{x}_2$ are the means from the samples 1 and 2.
Degrees of freedom (df) = $(n_1-1) + (n_2-1)$.

Degrees of freedom (df)

- Are the number of items that can be varied in relation to the other items. If there is only one item it cannot be varied in relation to another so there are 0 degrees of freedom.
- Used in preference to sample size.
- Equals the number of observation − 1 $(n-1)$.

Non-parametric tests. Also known as distribution free statistical tests. Used when:
- Data are **qualitative**.
  - Measured by
    - Nominal
    - Ordinal (rank) scale.
- Data are not **normally** distributed.
- Data **distribution** is unknown.
  Can be used for parametric data but not as powerful as specific parametric tests.
Makes no assumptions about the underlying distribution of the sample.
- Can be used on small samples.

13. Chi-square (χ^2) test is suitable for:
   - Nominal and ordinal data.
   - The test compares the frequency of observed results against the frequency that would be expected, as if there was NO difference between the two groups.

$$\chi^2 = \frac{\text{sum of (observed − expected)}^2}{\text{expected}}$$

   - P value is determined by checking calculated χ^2 in table against degrees of freedom.
   - A larger χ^2 value, the smaller the probability P.

Example of a Chi-squared test

100 Patients are given 7 mg atracurium before suxamethonium and 100 patients are only given suxamethonium. They are described as either in pain or pain-free from suxamethonium pains.

If the atracurium has no effect, then an equal proportion in each group will have pain.

If significantly fewer people experience pain then we conclude that the two groups are not statistically the same presumable because of the effect of the atracurium.

Contingency Table

	Painful	Pain free
Without atracurium	90 expected (E)	10
With atracurium	40 observed (O)	60
Observed – expected	40–90	60–10
$(0 - E)$	–50	+50
$(0 - E)^2$	2500	2500
$\dfrac{(0 - E)^2}{t}$	$\dfrac{2500}{90}$	$\dfrac{2500}{10}$

$$\text{Total } \frac{(0 - E)^2}{t} = 26 + 250 = 276$$

The Chi^2 value of 276 is then compared against the degrees of freedom on tables to give a P value of significance.

The number of degrees of freedom in a Chi-squared test is the number of columns – 1 multiplied by the number of rows – 1 or $(2–1) \times (2–1) = 1$.

- Chi-squared test is used to measure change in actual numbers of occurrence and NOT percentages, or other derived statistics.
- It is used for actual readings or measurements and not derived statistics.

Yates correction factor
- Used for small samples to decrease the Chi-squared value.

Wilcoxon rank sum test is suitable for:
- Ordinal data
- Unpaired data.

Can substitute for paired 't' test.

Wilcoxon signed rank test is suitable for:
- Matched data
- Paired data.

Can replace the two sample "t" test.

Mann–Whitney test
■ Extends the Wilcoxon test to handle groups of unequal numbers.
■ Can be used when the data are interval, continuous or ratio that are not normally distributed.

Kruskal–Wallis test:
■ Can be used when the data are interval, continuous, ratio type that are not normally distributed.
■ When more than two groups of data are involved.

Fisher's exact probability test:
■ Used when the frequency in any one cell of the contingency table is less than 5.
■ Used when result is YES or NO.

14. Correlation or association. This is the **strength** of the relationship between two variables. Plotted as a scattergram of X against Y.
    ■ Called the correlation coefficient (r) or Pearson's product moment correlation coefficient.
    ■ Value from −1 to +1.
    ■ A value near 1 means the relationship is significant or strong.

Correlation coefficient (r) + or − value	Degree of association
1	Complete
0.8–1.0	Strong
0.5–0.8	Moderate
0.2–0.5	Weak
0–0.2	Negligible
0	None

Positive (+) a rise in one linked to a rise in the other.
Negative (−) a rise in one linked to a fall in the other.
Horizontal line is no correlation.

Graphs of relationships
Spearman's and Kendall's rank correlation coefficients are non parametric alternatives to Pearson's correlation coefficient.

Linear regression (see graphs opposite)
■ Mainly used when there is one measured dependent variable (X) and one or more independent variable(s) (Y).
■ Multiple regression predicts a single dependent variable against a number of independent variables.
■ Y is a random variable.
■ Y is a dependent variable in a linear regression.
Formula for the line:

$$Y = alpha\ (\alpha) + beta\ (\beta)\ X$$

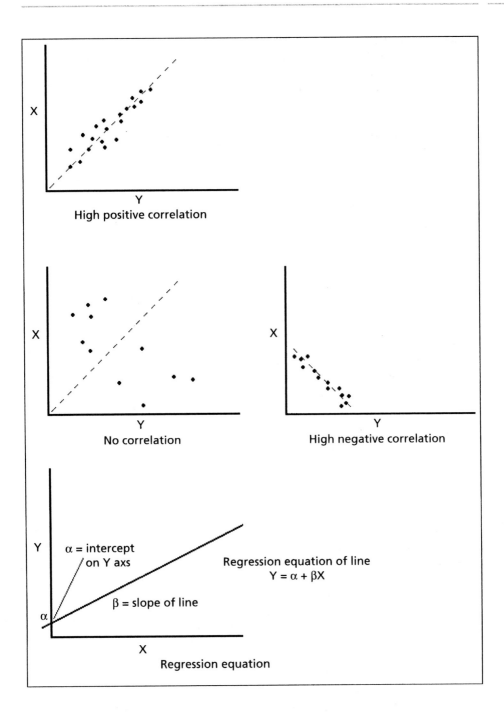

High positive correlation

No correlation

High negative correlation

α = intercept on Y axs

Regression equation of line
Y = α + βX

β = slope of line

Regression equation

where:

- X is an independent variable capable of measurement without an error
- α alpha is a parameter, the value of Y when X = 0 or the intercept on the y axis.
- β beta is the regression coefficient and measures the "slope of the line", i.e. the change in Y per unit increase in X.

Self-test 1: Propofol study *(Answers on page 361)*

An anaesthetist records the dose of propofol required to induce anaesthesia in her patient and the time it takes for a patient to become unresponsive to a painful stimulus. The anaesthetist repeats this on nine more patients and then uses thiopentone on 10 more patients.

The doses of propofol in mg were: 100, 110, 120, 150, 150, 160, 160, 160, 160, 200.

The doses of thiopentone in mg were: 150, 150, 200, 200, 200, 250, 250, 300, 300, 500.

Questions

1. What words best describe these data: qualitative, quantitative, variable?

2. When the results for propofol dosage are plotted against the number of patients:
   a. There will be a normal distribution curve
   b. The curve will be bimodal
   c. The degree of variation will be given by the mode, median and mean.

3. The mode result for propofol is 160.

4. There are a number of inadequacies in this study if meaningful deductions are to be made from these figures. What are they?

5. The standard deviation for the dose of propofol includes:
   a. 33.3%
   b. 66.6%
   c. 99.9% of the results.

6. The anaesthetist wishes to compare the doses of each drug with the time to recovery of each patient. Is there likely to be a negative correlation?

7. The value of r for the correlation between two sets of results is −1, what does this mean?
   a. No correlation
   b. Mistake in the calculations
   c. Good positive correlation
   d. Perfect negative correlation.

8. The results suggest that there is no bias in the study. True or False?

9. To double the precision of the study there would need to be:
   a. 40 patients
   b. 80 patients
   c. 100 patients
   d. 400 patients.

10. The probability of something never happening is represented by the number

    a. 1

    b. 2

    c. 0

    d. −1.

11. For medical purposes if a result lies outside one standard deviation we say this has a probability of 0.05 and is unlikely to occur by chance. True or False?

An anaesthetist is interested in how much pain is caused by an injection of propofol and so decides to randomly allocate patients to receive either propofol or thiopentone and then to ask them afterwards if the site of injection is painful, or if the arm is painful.

With propofol, 20 out of 25 patients said the site was painful and 10 out of 25 said the arm was painful.

With thiopentone, 5 said the site was painful and 0 said the arm was painful.

Questions

1. These data are:
  a. Quantitative
  b. Continuous
  c. Not analysable statistically
  d. Non-parametric data.

2. It is appropriate to use the Wilcoxon matched pairs test.   True   False

3. Before performing a Chi-squared test, a contingency table would be:

	Pain	No pain	Total
Propofol	20	5	25
Thiopentone	5	20	25
Total	25	25	50

True   False

4. Expected observations would be:

	Pain	No pain	Total
Propofol	12.5	12.5	25
Thiopentone	12.5	12.5	25
Total	25	25	50

True   False

5. An appropriate null hypothesis would be that intravenous injections are always painful.   True   False

6. Chi-squared for these results is:
  a. 4.24
  b. 5.76
  c. 6.86.

7. There are 3 degrees of freedom.   True   False

8. The data suitable for a Chi-squared analysis are:
  a. Random.

b. Quantitative data.

c. Values in excess of 1.

9. The following measurements are made preoperatively on 100 patients:
   a. Haemoglobin concentrations.
   b. Arterial oxygen saturation.
   c. Serum creatinine concentrations.

Draw a distribution curve for each and explain how they differ.

Answers – Self-test 1: Propofol study

1. These results are measured and therefore quantitative. Qualitative data involves group numbers, ratios and percentages. Any measured data, which varies, is a variable.

2. *a.* Normally distributed, bell-shaped or Gaussian distribution.
   b. Strictly speaking, the curve will not be a true bell-shaped curve but will probably have more results in the lower range compared to the upper range. This observation applies to many analgesic and hypnotic drugs.
   c. Mean, mode and median are measures of the central values. Variation is given by the standard deviation and the variance.

3. Mode is the most frequently occurring number. Mean is the total divided by the number of results or average. Median is the middle number in rank order.

4. It would have been better to have randomised the patients to receive either treatment A or B. If they came for a second GA then the treatments could have been crossed over, as might happen in ECT. It was not double blind. Doses are not expressed according to weight. Inadequate sample size. It is possible some patients were ill, receiving other drugs, or had illness, which may have affected the doses so exclusion criteria need to be clearly stated.

5. *b.* – 66.6%.
   The mean is 157, subtract each value from the mean and sum them gives 200. Square 200 and divide by $n-1$. Then take the square root for the SD.

6. No. If there is a correlation it will be positive with these results. The dose increases as the time to recovery increases.

7. *d.* – A figure of 1 is a perfect correlation. Any result less than -1 or greater than $+1$ would be impossible.

8. **False** – Bias is a measure of how close the extreme figures are from the average. In this case there are doses away from the mean or average dose. This could be explained by different weights of patients.

9. Precision is the degree to which all the doses are close together. A measure of precision is n/rho.

   To double the precision the sample number needs to be multiplied by 4: $20 \times 4 = 80$.

10. Probability ranges from 0 = never or impossible happening to +1 always or inevitable happening.

11. **False** – The result must lie outside 95% of the results. That is in the 2.5% at both extremes, above and below. 1 standard deviation will include about 68% and two standard deviations 95% of readings.

Answers – Self-test 2: Propofol pain

1. These are qualitative data; the data are not continuous but can be analysed statistically; i.e. non-parametric data.

2. **False.** The Wilcoxon matched-pairs signed-rank test requires that measurements are made. A second set of measurements is made and the difference between the first and second reading calculated. These differences are then put in a rank order starting with the least or most negative difference. The results are ranked in order of magnitude. This test is equivalent to the Student's *t*-test for parametric data.

3. **True.**

4. **True** – Expected results = row total × column total/grand total.

5. **False** – The null hypothesis would be that both drugs cause pain equally.

6. Chi-squared = total of O – E/E.
   This works out as O – E/E = 0.6 (4 observations). So, sum is 2.4, squared 5.76.

7. **False** – Degrees of freedom = rows –1 × columns – 1 = 1.
   There is one degree of freedom. In a 2 × 2 table, once one figure has been set, all the others follow from the totals.

8. Criteria: random, qualitative, no expected frequency less than 5.

9. *a.* Haemoglobin concentrations will be normally distributed.
   b. Arterial oxygen saturation will be negatively skewed. No patient can have more than 100% and many will have 97–100% but there will be a tail of lower results.
   c. Creatinine concentrations will show a positive skewed curve. Most people will have low creatinine concentrations but some will have elevated levels.

X-RAYS

12

Anaesthetists should be familiar with plain films of the chest, skull, neck and lumbar spine. Lung scans. CT and MRI scans of the head, neck, thorax, abdomen and spine. Cardiac echocardiogram and coronary angiograms.

Plain film of the chest

Check:
- PA or AP. AP films are portable and because the beam comes from in front the anterior structures such as the heart will be magnified. PA films have the scapulae out of the lung field and the clavicles lower in the chest (see Figure below)
- Exposure.
  - Normal – The upper thoracic vertebrae should be visible down to about T6.
  - Over-exposure – More vertebrae seen.
  - Under-exposure – Fewer vertebrae seen.
  Good and bad films are not helpful terms.

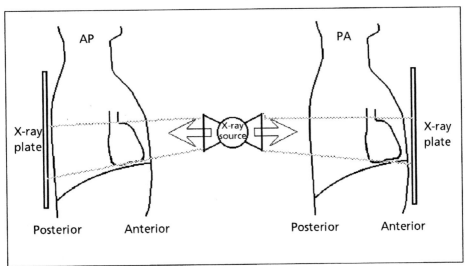

Anterior–posterior and posterior–anterior radiography

▪ Rotation. The sternal ends of the clavicle should be equal distances from the vertebral spines. There should be no parallax of the vertebrae.

System for examining the film

a. Mediastinum

Look at trachea – central and width of airway. Position of carina should be at about T6.

b. Heart shadow

To right of mediastinum right atrium; to the left aorta, left atrium and left ventricle. The left hilum is slightly higher than the right.

c. Lung fields

Diaphragm, the left is lower than the right – any change may guide towards the side of abnormality. Normally, six anterior and eight posterior ribs should be seen, more with horizontal position indicates hyperinflation.

Rotate the film through 90° to the side to see a pneumothorax, rotate through 180° to examine the bony structures – ribs for fractures and soft tissues for air.

d. The spine

Cervical spine in extension and flexion. Look for the line of the anterior and posterior vertebral bodies, the posterior boundary of the vertebral canal and the posterior boundary of the spines. The distance from the axis to the odontoid peg is normally 2 mm.

e. Lumbar spine

Look for the normal lumbar curves and, as in the cervical region, the lines of the anterior and posterior vertebral bodies and the spinous processes.

On the AP film, the interpedicular distance taken between the medial borders of the pedicles is the maximum width of the spinal canal. This distance will normally be 25–30 mm getting larger from L1 to L5. If the distance varies by more than 2 mm between vertebrae there is an abnormal erosion or enlargement. The shortest vertical distance between the pedicles is a measure of the height of the intervertebral foramen. It also indicates the height of the disc spaces, which normally increase from the upper to the lower lumbar region. Narrowing commonly occurs with osteophytes from the vertebral bodies or the zygoapophyseal joints

On a lateral film, a line from the posterior body of the vertebral body to the spino-laminar line should be 18 mm. Less than 15 mm is evidence of stenosis.

X-ray 1 *(Answers on page 399)*

The chest X-rays in the examination hall will be full size X-rays with identification marks removed. For reproduction in black and white we have used computer-generated chest X-rays for these examples.

Questions

1. This chest X-ray is an AP film.	True	False
2. The film is over-exposed.	True	False
3. The heart is enlarged.	True	False
4. Interstitial lines or Kerley B lines are present.	True	False
5. The right border of the heart on the X-ray is the right ventricle.	True	False
6. The patient should be managed as if he has a fixed cardiac output.	True	False

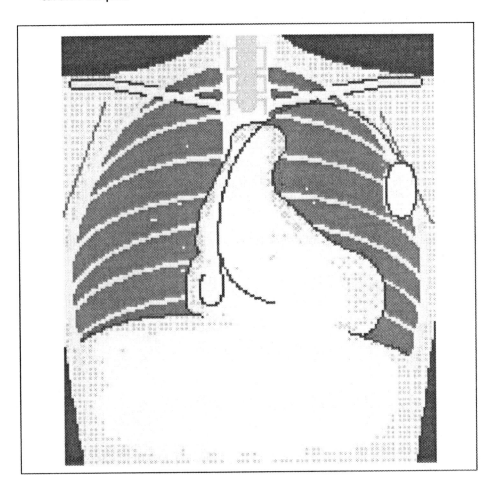

7. One pacemaker wire is in the right atrium.   True   False

8. One of the pacemaker electrodes will be a sensing
   electrode.   True   False

9. The patient should receive preoperative antibiotics.   True   False

10. Bipolar diathermy will be safer than unipolar diathermy.   True   False

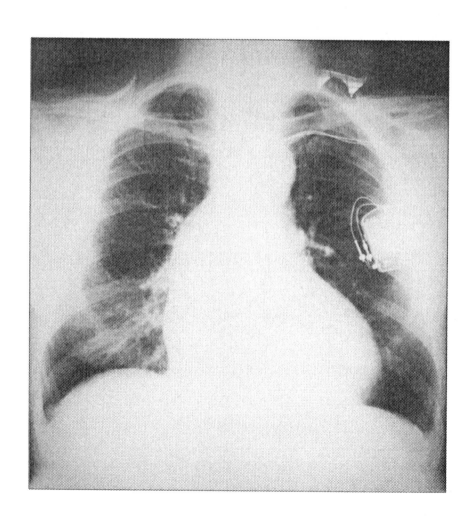

X-ray 2 *(Answers on page 400)*

Questions

1. This chest X-ray is a PA film.   True   False

2. The left border of the heart from above downwards is
   the aortic arch, pulmonary vessels, left atrium and the
   right ventricle.   True   False

3. The left lung field is normal.   True   False

4. The diaphragms are normal.   True   False

5. The left atrium is enlarged.   True   False

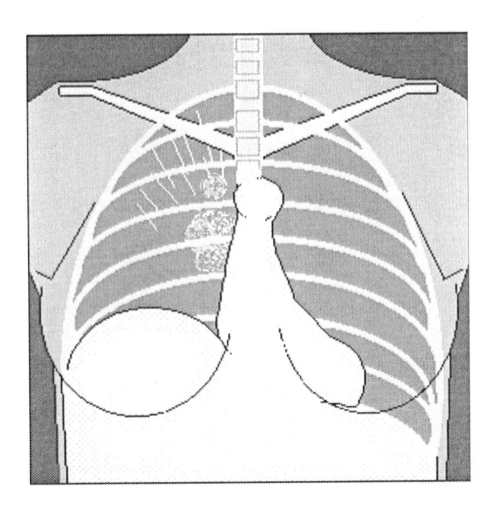

6. The patient has probably been a cigarette smoker.   True   False

7. The patient could have at least two nerve palsies.   True   False

8. The patient might complain of hoarseness.   True   False

9. The patient has either had tuberculosis or has been
   treated for their lung condition.   True   False

10. A bone scan should be performed before considering
    a bronchoscopy.   True   False

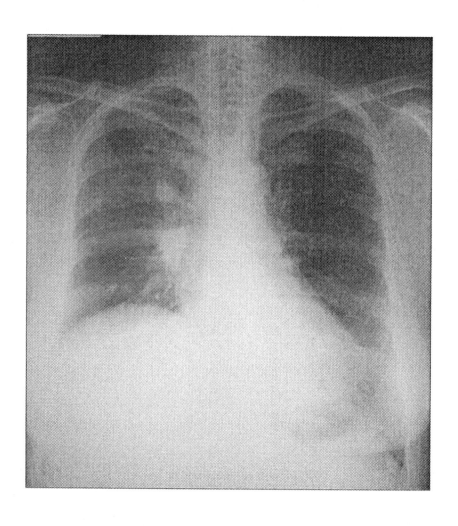

X-ray 3 *(Answers on page 401)*

Questions

1. This chest X-ray is an AP film.   True   False

2. The heart is enlarged.   True   False

3. The film has been taken in deep inspiration.   True   False

4. The film is over-penetrated.   True   False

5. The patient is likely to have had chest pain.   True   False

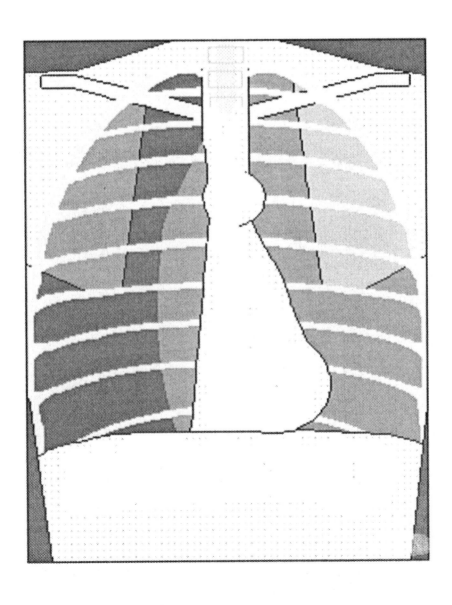

6. The patient's cardiac output will be impaired.   True   False

7. The administration of Entonox will increase the cardiac
   output.   True   False

8. Intubation and ventilation may increase the cardiac
   output.   True   False

9. The left lung is hyperinflated.   True   False

10. Tetracycline injected into the intra-pleural space may
    have a place in the management of this patient.   True   False

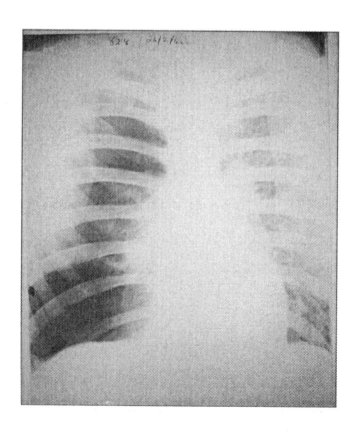

X-Ray 4 *(Answers on page 402)*

Questions
1. The X-ray is reasonably centred.   True   False

2. The film is of normal penetration.   True   False

3. The left lung is hyperinflated.   True   False

4. The trachea is dilated.   True   False

5. The patient is at risk from aspiration.   True   False

6. The patient may have an associated iron deficiency anaemia.   True   False

7. Cricoid pressure will be effective.   True   False

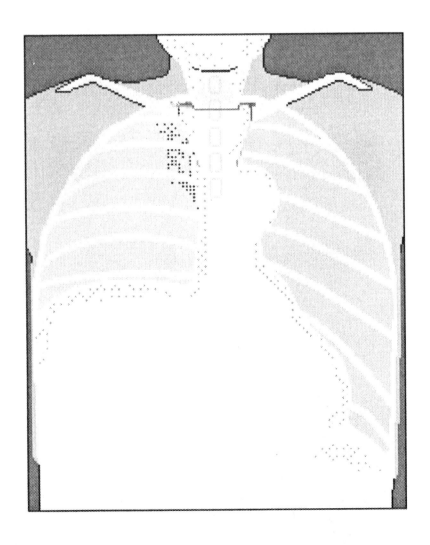

8. The patient needs chest physiotherapy.　　True　False

9. An inhalation induction is indicated if the patient requires a general anaesthetic.　　True　False

10. A nasogastric tube will pass easily.　　True　False

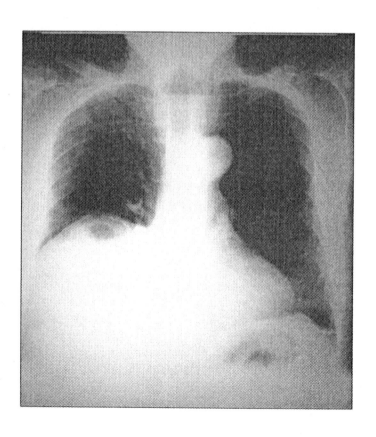

X-Ray 5

(Answers on page 403)

Questions

1. It would be reasonable to take this X-ray at any time. True False

2. This is a PA film. True False

3. The film is taken in deep inspiration. True False

4. There is evidence of left atrial enlargement. True False

5. Interstitial lines or Kerley B lines are present. True False

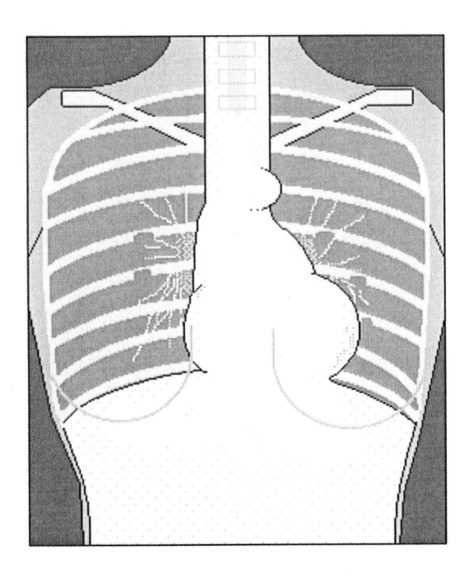

6. In this patient the blood pressure will be abnormal.   True   False

7. Pulmonary oedema is present.   True   False

8. The patient might have Turner's syndrome.   True   False

9. The patient will probably have a bicuspid aortic valve.   True   False

10. The patient may need treatment for hypertension.   True   False

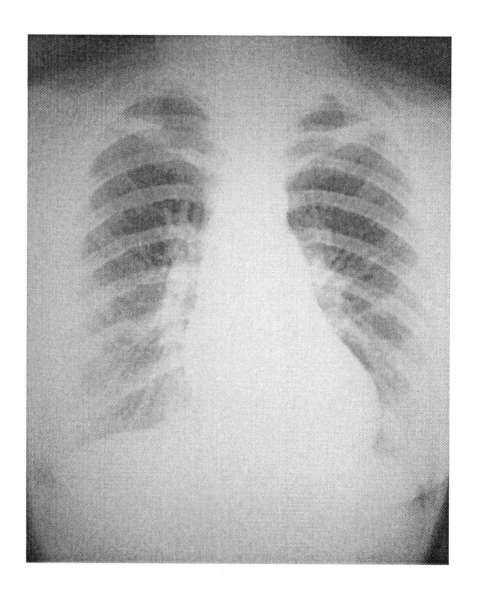

X-Ray 6

(Answers on page 404)

Questions

1. This is an AP film.		True	False
2. The film is over-penetrated.		True	False
3. The right lung field is over-inflated.		True	False
4. There is a left pleural effusion.		True	False
5. A specimen of sputum should be obtained for culture.		True	False
6. The patient may be symptom-free.		True	False

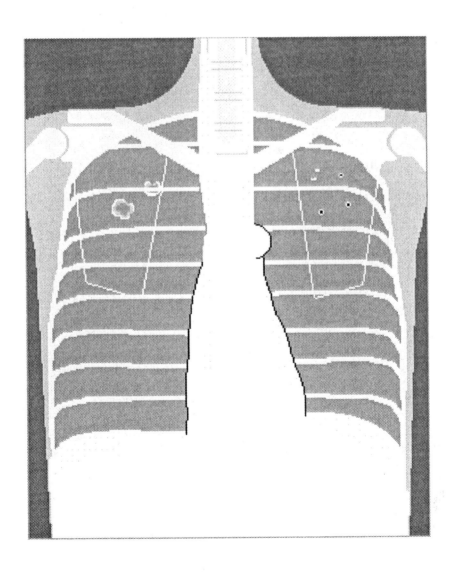

7. If no sputum is available a fibreoptic bronchoscopy should be performed. True False

8. The patient will have an increased total lung capacity. True False

9. Intubation and ventilation may lead to reduced oxygenation. True False

10. This patient should have their α1-antitrypsin assayed in the serum. True False

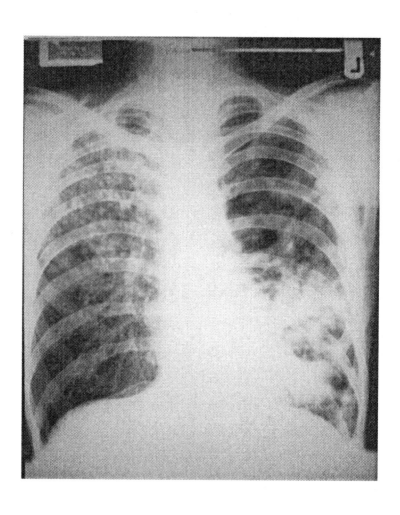

X-ray 7 *(Answers on page 405)*

Echocardiogram
The echo can be a 2-D mode or an M-mode.

The diagram shows: Upper 2-D and lower m-mode parasternal echocardiogram with a schematic representation alongside.

Questions
1. On the 2-D mode what are the parts labelled A to D?

2. What is abnormal about C on the echo?

3. From the M-mode trace, what are the features labelled E , F and G

4. What can be learnt from the trace at H?

5. What is the ejection fraction?

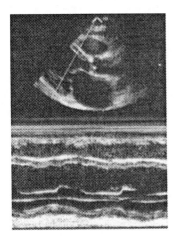

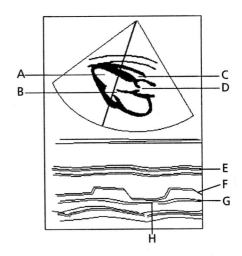

X-Ray 8

(Answers on page 406)

Questions

1. What is the figure below?

2. What apparatus is used?

3. What agents are used to give this picture?

4. What does this show?

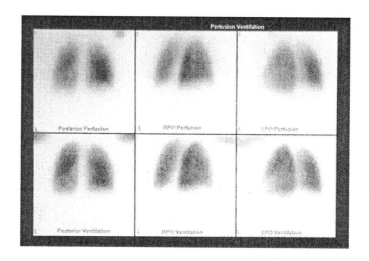

X-ray 9

(Answers on page 407)

Cervical spine
Questions
1. Which view of the cervical spine is shown below?

2. How many vertebrae should be seen on a good film?

3. Why is it important to take more than one x-ray of this view?

4. What is indicated by the following lines: a, b, c, d, e, f, g?

5. What should lines c–f be like?

6. Name three conditions in which excessive movement of the axis on the atlas may occur.

7. There is some irregularity of the anterior vertebral bodies. To what is this due?

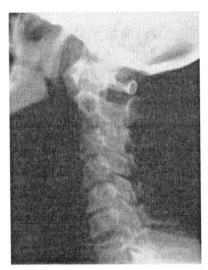
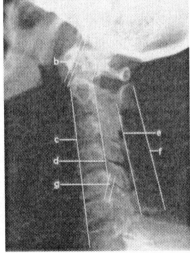

X-ray 10

(Answers on page 408)

Lumbar spine

Questions

1. What are the two X-rays shown on this and the following page of?

2. How many lumbar vertebrae are normally present?

3. What are the normal parts of a lumbar vertebra?

4. What are the normal and abnormal curves seen on examination of a lumbar X-ray. What may changes from the normal mean?

5. How is the size of the spinal canal assessed with reference to lines a, b and c on the pictures?

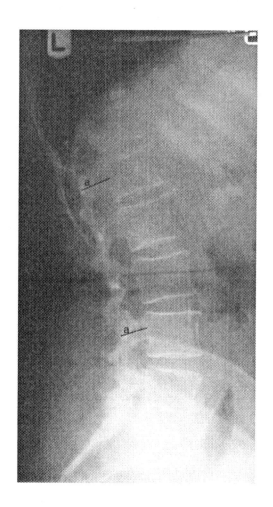

6. How is narrowing of the intervertebral foramen assessed and what common condition causes narrowing?

7. What are the differences between the zygoapophyseal joints of the lumbar region compared to those in the cervical region?

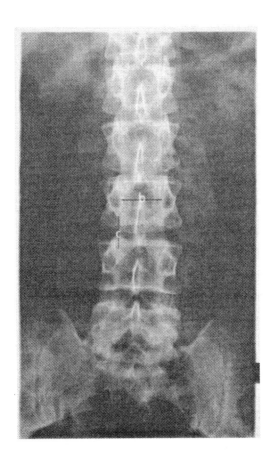

X-ray 11 (Answers on page 409)

Head and neck

Questions

1. What is the main feature in picture A?

2. What is the main feature in picture B?

3. What other features might be present on X-ray and illustrated here?

4. What signs and symptoms may be present?

5. What is the normal history of lesion A?

6. What is the normal history of lesion B?

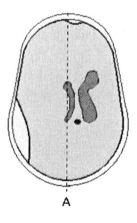

A

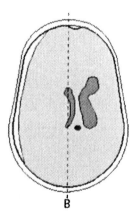

B

Self-tests

Use each of the following 14 X-rays to practice a technique of examination. Each of these X-rays shows a significant abnormality. What is it and what relevance, if any, does it have for the anaesthetists?

Self-test 1

(Answers on page 410)

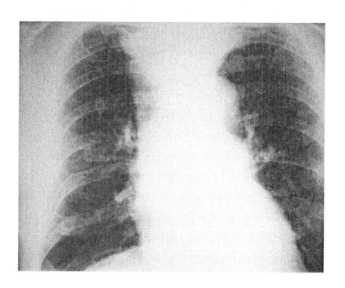

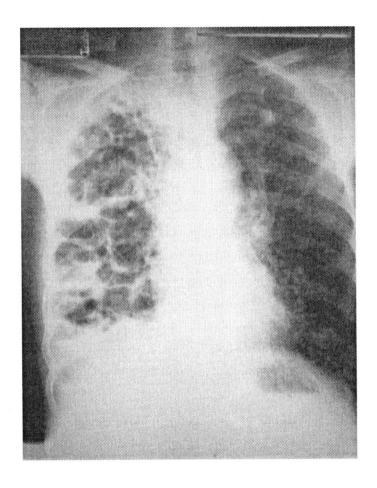

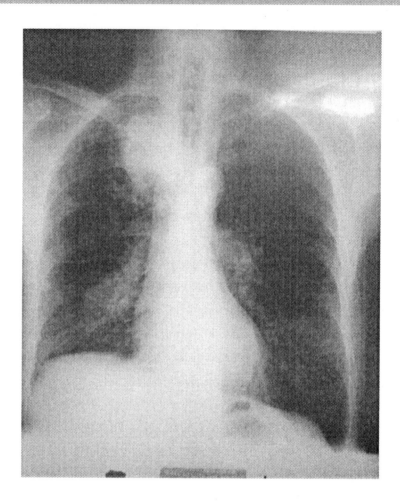

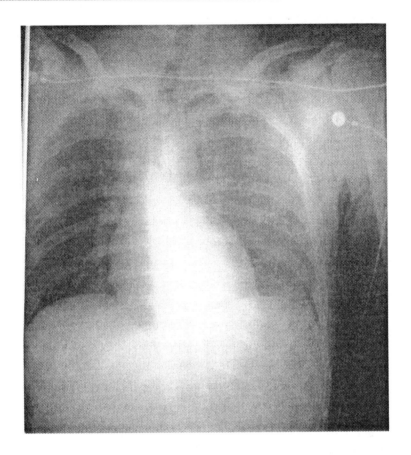

Self-test 5

(Answers on page 410)

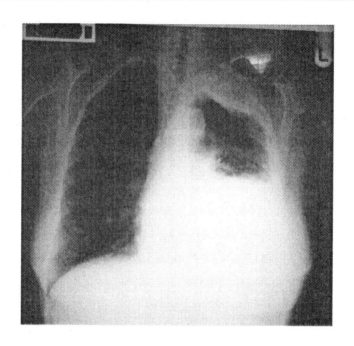

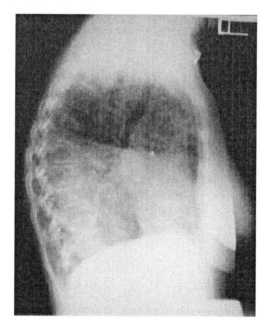

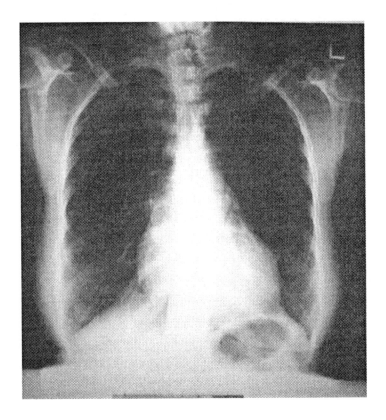

Self-test 7 (Answers on page 410)

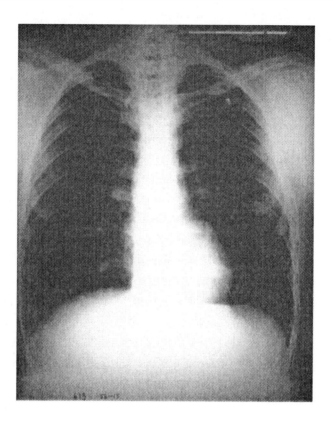

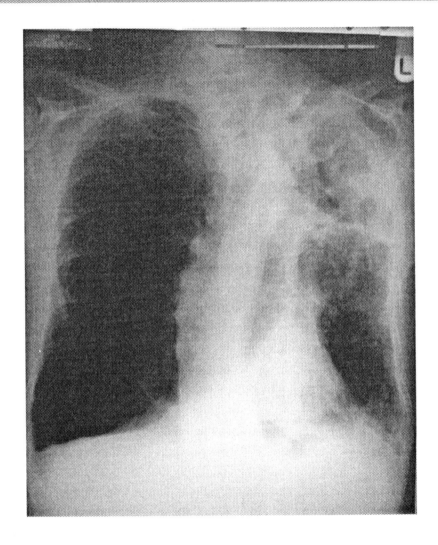

Self-test 9

(Answers on page 411)

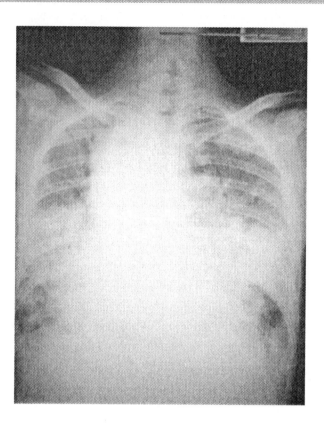

Self-test 10

(Answers on page 411)

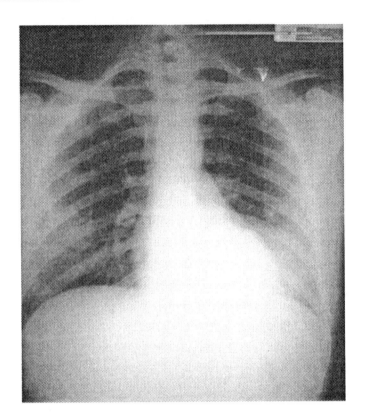

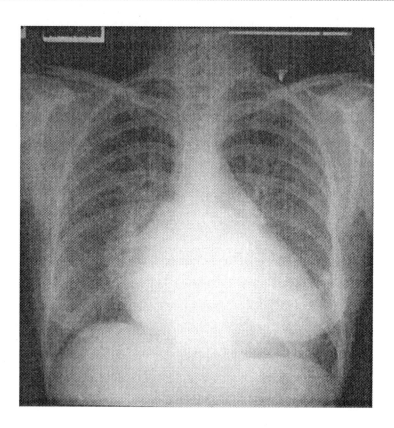

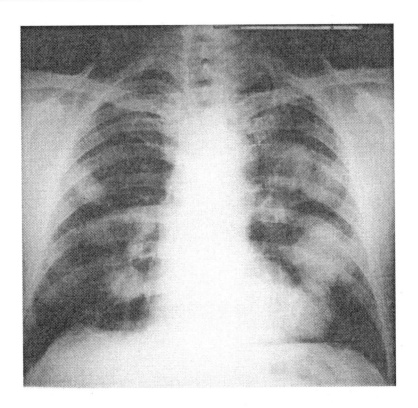

Self-test 13 (Answers on page 411)

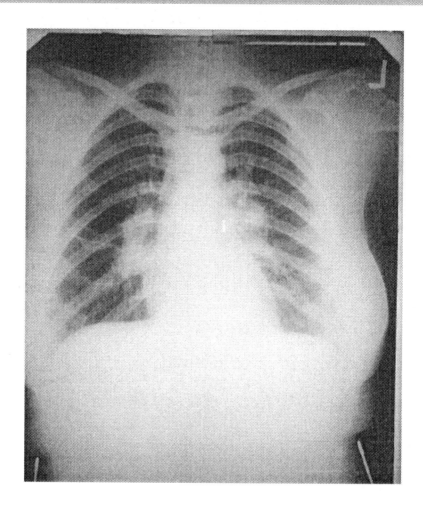

Self-test 14

(Answers on page 411)

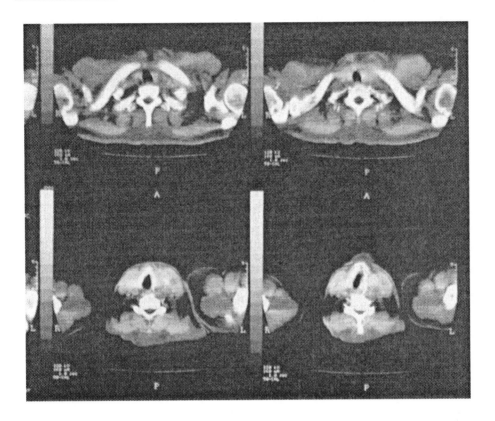

Answers
X-rays

Answers – X-ray 1

1. False – The scapula have been rotated out of the lung fields. The X-ray should be labelled.

2. False – The vertebral bodies are poorly seen in the upper thoracic region, indicating under penetration. If the vertebral bodies are seen to about T4, then this is normal penetration. If more are seen through the cardiac shadow then this is over penetration. It is suggested that referring to this as good and bad penetration does not mean a great deal. Penetration is important in assessing the density of the lung fields.

3. True – The diameter of the heart shadow is over half the diameter of the thorax.

4. False.

5. False – It is the right atrium.

6. True – Old pacemakers are fixed-rate. New pacemakers may respond to physiological changes but there may still be limited myocardial function.

7. True.

8. True – Where two electrodes exist, one will be sensing.

9. False – The presence of a pacemaker is not an indication for prophylactic antibiotics.

10. True – Bipolar diathermy limits the field of spread of current. Unipolar diathermy is safe if the current field is over 15 cm from any part of the device, and there is no break in the insulation of the device.

Summary
The X-ray shows a pacemaker with two electrode leads; one fixed in the right atrium and the second in the right ventricle. The heart is enlarged.

Answers – X-ray 2

1. **True** – The scapula have been rotated out of the lung fields.

2. **False** – Below the pulmonary vessels and hilum is the left atrium and then the left ventricle.

3. **True.**

4. **False** – The right diaphragm is significantly elevated. If the lung is collapsed there might also be a reduction in the intercostal spaces and a shift in the mediastinum. An elevated hemi-diaphragm may also be due to an enlarged liver, if on the right, or a phrenic crush.

5. **False** – Signs of left atrial enlargement are: enlargement of the left atrial appendage on the left border of the heart and a double contour within the heart shadow.

6. **True** – There is a carcinoma at the right hilum. Primary lung carcinoma is more likely to occur in a smoker than in a non smoker. Secondary carcinoma may be from carcinoma of the breast, thyroid, kidney or prostate.

7. **True** – Phrenic and recurrent laryngeal nerve palsies.

8. **True** – This patient complained of hoarseness due to recurrent laryngeal nerve palsy. The left recurrent laryngeal nerve curves around the remnant of the ductus arteriosus. The right recurrent laryngeal nerve curves around the right subclavian artery. Because the left nerve has been drawn further into the chest than the right, it is more often affected by intrathoracic disease.

9. **True** – There is right apical fibrosis. The commonest cause of upper lobe fibrosis is tuberculosis, another cause may be following radiotherapy.

10. **False** – Not unless the patient complains of symptoms such as bone pain.

Answers – X-ray 3

1. **True** – The scapula are within the lung fields. This is not always a reliable sign as some patients may have difficulty in rotating their shoulders.

2. **False** – The cardiac diameter is within half of the diameter of the thorax.

3. **True** – The diaphragms are flat as in deep inspiration but this is also a feature of emphysema or a tension pneumothorax.

4. **False** – The film is under penetrated as the vertebrae cannot be seen in the upper thoracic region.

5. **True** – Due to the left pneumothorax.

6. **False** – This does not appear as a tension pneumothorax at present. The trachea and mediastinum are central.

7. **True** – Nitrous oxide will enter the pneumothorax faster than nitrogen will be displaced out due to the higher solubility of nitrous oxide. In a short period, the 50% oxygen and the relief of any pain from the Entonox will improve oxygenation but the increased size of the pneumothorax may reduce cardiac output.

8. **False** – Ventilation may create a tension pneumothorax.

9. **True** – There are at least nine ribs which are horizontal and widely spaced. This is to be expected with a pneumothorax. The X-ray findings are often complicated by an increased blood flow in the opposite lung to compensate for the reduced blood flow in the affected lung.

10. **True** – If the lung does not expand, then tetracycline mixed with local anaesthetic can be used to produce a chemical pleurodesis. It has the advantage of not being as painful as either talc or an open pleurodesis.

Answers – X-ray 4

1. True – The medial ends of the clavicles appear symmetrically placed in relationship to the sternum and the spines of the cervical vertebrae.

2. True – The vertebral bodies can be seen to about T4.

3. False – There are not more than eight ribs visible posteriorly.

4. False.

5. True – There is a fluid level in the upper mediastinum. This is diagnostic of an upper oesophageal obstruction or a pouch.

6. True – This could be an upper oesophageal web associated with Plummer–Vinson syndrome – glossitis and anaemia.

7. False – The pouch takes its origin above the cricoid: from the oesophagus, between the upper (thyropharyngeus) and the lower (cricopharyngeus) parts of the inferior constrictor.

8. True – There is evidence of right lung collapse, probably as a result of inhalation from the pouch. On the right the diaphragm is elevated and the ribs are close together.

9. True – This is an anaesthetic dilemma. The use of local anaesthetic and awake/fibreoptic intubation might be another alternative.

10. False – A nasogastric tube might coil up in the pouch, come back into the mouth or pass into the stomach.

Answers – X-ray 5

1. **False** – This is a female patient who should not be X-rayed in early pregnancy unless absolutely essential.

2. **True** – The scapula have been abducted, the clavicles are tilted and, if visible, the 1st rib would be tilted.

3. **True** – The diaphragms are low and flat in a PA film.

4. **True** – The left atrial border is more prominent.

5. **False** – Interstitial lines or Kerley B lines indicate interstitial oedema.

6. **True** – There is erosion of the undersurface of the ribs, indicating a possible coarctation. The notching usually affects the 4th to 8th ribs. The blood pressure will be higher in the right arm than in the legs.

7. **False.**

8. **True** – There is an association between coarctation and Turner's syndrome.

9. **True** – 80% of patients with a coarctation have bicuspid and later stenotic aortic valves.

10. **True** – Older patients with coarctation develop hypertension as a result of reduced renal perfusion.

Answers – X-ray 6

1. **True** – The scapula are covering the lung fields.

2. **False** – The film is under-penetrated as vertebral bodies cannot be seen below the clavicle.

3. **True** – The right lung fields are over-inflated as judged by the presence of more than eight ribs posteriorly or six ribs anteriorly. The appearance of the posterior ribs are horizontal and widely spaced, indicating emphysema.

4. **False** – None seen.

5. **True.**

6. **True** – It is possible to have pulmonary tuberculosis without symptoms.

7. **True** – Washings with a bronchoscope and biopsies are reliable means of making a diagnosis of active tuberculosis.

8. **True.**

9. **True** – If there is pulmonary hypertension. IPPV may severely limit cardiac output.

10. **True** – There is an inherited deficiency in 2% of emphysema patients, some will also have liver disease.

Answers – X-ray 7

1. **A** – Left ventricle
   B – Mitral valve
   C – Left atrium
   D – Aortic valve.

2. The left atrium is enlarged.

3. The trace shows E the intraventricular septum, F the anterior mitral valve cusp, G the posterior mitral valve cusp.

4. E shows the mitral valve leaflets or cusps coming together. In this trace there is poor movement of the posterior cups towards the transducer and poor movement of the anterior cusp, indicating stenosis. It appears that the cusps do not come together fully, indicating incompetence.

5. The ejection fraction is the stoke volume from the left ventricle as a percentage of the left ventricular volume.

Answers – X-ray 8

1. A normal lung scan.

2. A gamma camera.

3. Gamma-radiated thallium, attached to albumin with molecules of 20 micron size, is injected. The albumin ensures that the thallium 201 is concentrated in the lung circulation. The patient breathes radiated Krypton 81 gas.

4. This lung scan shows poorly perfused areas indicating a pulmonary embolism.

Answers – X-ray 9

1. Lateral – probably flexion.

2. All seven cervical vertebrae.

3. A flexion and extension view should be taken to show if there is excessive movement of the odontoid in the axis.

4. a. The odontoid peg.
   b. The distance between the odontoid and the axis – normally 2 mm, can be up to 5 mm.
   c. The anterior border of the vertebral bodies.
   d. The line of the posterior vertebral bodies.
   e. Line of the posterior boundary of the vertebral canal.
   f. Line of the posterior boundary of the spines.
   g. An intervertebral zygo apophyseal joint (often wrongly called a facet joint). Note that the joints are anterior to the vertebral canal in the cervical vertebrae. This allows for greater rotation movement than elsewhere in the spine.

5. The lines c–f should all be smooth lines. Any irregularity is caused by disease, trauma or tumour.

6. Trauma, rheumatoid arthritis, Down's syndrome.

7. Osteoarthritis.

Answers – X-ray 10

1. Plain X-ray films, AP and lateral of the lumbar spine.

2. Five.

3. Body, pedicle and laminar surrounding the vertebral arch. Transverse processes attached to the junction of laminar and pedicle and spine attached to the laminar.

4. A normal AP position is straight, abnormal lateral curve – scoliosis. Normal lateral position shows a lordosis, abnormal loss of lordosis making the spine straight. Acute loss of the lumbar curve of lordosis with scoliosis due to muscle spasm is likely to indicate a disc herniation. Chronic loss of curves is associated with degenerative disease.

5. On an AP film, the inter-pedicle distance (line b), taken between the medial borders of the pedicles is the maximum width of the spinal canal. This distance will normally be 25–30 mm getting larger from L1 to L5.

The mean distance varies in an adult from 29 mm in the cervical region, 17 mm in the thoracic region to 26 mm in the lumbar region. In children, the mean distance will be 4 mm less in the neck and 5–6 mm less in the lumbar region.

If the distance varies by more than 2 mm between vertebrae there is an abnormal erosion or enlargement.

On a lateral film a line from the posterior body of the vertebral body to the spino-laminar line (line a) should be 18 mm. Less than 15 mm is evidence of stenosis.

6. The shortest vertical distance between the pedicles (line c) is a measure of the height of the intervertebral foramen. It also indicates the height of the disc spaces, which normally increase from the upper to the lower lumbar region.

Narrowing commonly occurs with osteophytes from the vertebral bodies or the zygoapophyseal joints.

7. The zygoapophyseal joints in the lumbar region lie posterior to the vertebral canal. The joint line lies in an anterior–posterior plane. There is little movement possible at these joints as the joint processes above wedge between the processes below.

The cervical joints lie just posterior to the cervical bodies and the joint line lies in a lateral plane. These joints are best placed for the rotation and extension–flexion movements between the cervical vertebrae.

Answers – X-ray 11

1. The picture A shows an extradural haematoma. This has a convex–convex outline.

2. The picture B shows a subdural haematoma.

3. The mid line may be shifted to the opposite side as judged by the position of the ventricles and the pineal body, which is calcified in adults. The ventricles may be reduced in size.

4. There may be clinical symptoms of raised intracranial pressure, head ache, vomiting, reduced consciousness. Signs of papilloedema, a 6th nerve palsy and unilateral weakness.

5. An extradural haematoma is due to arterial bleeding, e.g. from the middle meningial artery. It occurs within minutes of a head injury, which usually involves a skull fracture.

6. A subdural haematoma is due to tears in veins crossing the subdural space. It can present without a history of a head injury, increasing headache, confusion, and loss of consciousness. If there is a history of head injury it can be days before symptoms appear. There is usually no fracture.

Answer – Self-test 1

A superior mediastinal mass. There may be narrowing of the trachea and other airways. There may be SVC obstruction. A CT scan would help define the airway.

Answer – Self-test 2

Lung cysts. Nitrous oxide may expand the cysts and ventilation may also cause rupture. Each lung will have a different compliance. A double lumen tube and differential ventilation may be beneficial to avoid barotrauma and to ensure good oxygenation.

Answer – Self-test 3

An upper lobe mass. May cause recurrent nerve palsy or Horner's syndrome.

Answer – Self-test 4

The left diaphragm is elevated, the trachea pushed to the right. The left lung field is denser. Turn to picture on its side. A left sided pneumothorax, probably developing tension.

Answer – Self-test 5

Left lower lobe infection.

Answer – Self-test 6

Marked deviation to the left of the trachea. Intubation may not be easy.

Answer – Self-test 7

Flattened diaphragms, horizontal ribs with expansion of the intercostal spaces. Over 8 ribs seen. The mediastinal shadow is long and thin. A typical hyper-inflated, emphysematous chest.

Answer – Self-test 8

Kyphoscolioisis. Each lung will have a different compliance and filling/emptying characteristics. A double lumen tube and differential ventilation will help oxygenation.

Answer – Self-test 9

A very wet lung with almost a bat's wing shadow. The heart diameter is enlarged. Pulmonary oedema.

Answer – Self-test 10

This is always a tricky diagnosis. The left diaphragm is elevated. There is a double shadow along the left border of the heart of left lower lobe collapse.

Answer – Self-test 11

This is another straight left border of the heart. The heart is enlarged, particularly to the right of the mediastinum. The heart of mitral stenosis.

Answer – Self-test 12

These shadows are dense. Multiple tumours. Rounded in shape. Typical of cannon ball metastases

Answer – Self-test 13

Bilateral hilar masses of lymph nodes. These are from sarcoidosis.

Answer – Self-test 14

CT of neck. The trachea and larynx are compressed and deviated to the right. There is a tumour of the neck either thyroid or from lymphoid tissue. Difficult intubation.

ELECTROCARDIOGRAM 13

Examine the ECG methodically. Make a diagnosis of all the findings.

Calibration
Look for the rectangular pulse that should be a horizontal deflection of 0.5 cm for 0.2 seconds and a vertical deflection of 1 cm high for 1 millivolt.

Axis
- The normal axis is −30 to +90.
- Determine the axis from:
  - *a.* The main QRS above the isoelectric line points to the plane of the axis.
  - *b.* The lead with most negative QRS is at 180° to the axis.
  - *c.* The lead with equal area of QRS above and below the isoelectric line is at right angles to the axis.
- Left axis deviation in: abdominal masses pushing the diaphragm up, LVF, cardiomyopathy and LBBB.
- Right axis RVH, cor pulmonale, RBBB.

Rate
Rhythm strip. One small horizontal square is 0.04 seconds; one large square is 0.2 seconds.

Calculate rate by counting the number of large squares between two QRS complexes and dividing into 300:300 because there are 300 large squares of 0.2 second each in 60 seconds. Irregular pulse rate. Take a number of beats and divide the number of large squares into 300 × the number of beats.

Rhythm
PR interval normal < 0.2 seconds. Exclude an abnormal rhythm: irregular atrial fibrillation −no P wave, flutter P waves 2 or 3 to each QRS. Note a pacing spike. Longer PR in first degree heart block, link P to QRS and exclude other heart block.

P wave
Peaked with pulmonary hypertension, large right atrium.
M-shaped in mitral valve disease, large left atrium.

QRS

- < 0.12 seconds.
- *ST segment*: Reverse tick in digoxin therapy.
  - Elevated ischaemia.
  - Depressed infarction.
- *T wave*: > 5 mm hyperkalaemia.
- *QT interval*: Short digoxin therapy, hypercalcaemia.
  - Long hypocalcaemia, hypokalaemia, hypothermia, myocarditis.

Myocardial infarction

First change ST segment elevation. Second change within 48 hours.
Pathological Q wave. Third change, in days ST segment returns to normal.
Pathological Q wave >0.04 seconds, depth is not so important. Normal Q is <0.04 sec wide, <25% of the QRS height.

- Anterior – pathological Q in V1–3.
- Lateral – pathological Q in V4–6.
- Inferior – pathological Q in leads II and III.

Cardiac abnormalities

- *LVH.* Left axis deviation, the largest R in V5 or 6 and the largest S in V1 > 35 mm, ST depression, T wave inversion.
- *RVH.* Right axis deviation, P pulmonale, tall R waves in V1–2, or R: S ratio >1 in V1–2, T wave inversion in right sided chest leads V1–3, ST depression.
- RBBB spread of the electrical depolarisation into the right ventricle is delayed, QRS long, end S in lead 1, end R in V1.
- LBBB wide QRS complex in chest leads.
- Pulmonary embolism acute S in I, Q in III, T in III.
- *Pericarditis.* Steep curved ST elevation chest leads.
- *Wolf–Parkinson–White syndrome.* Type A: positive delta wave V1–6, negative delta lead I. Type B: biphasic or negative delta wave in V1–3, positive delta lead I.

ECG 1

(Answers on page 425)

Questions

1. The speed of this ECG is 0.5 cm/s.   True   False

2. The axis is within normal limits.   True   False

3. There is evidence that the patient might complain of angina.   True   False

4. There is second degree heart block (Mobitz 1).   True   False

5. There is right bundle branch block.   True   False

6. The patient is likely to have a serum potassium of 7 mmol/l.   True   False

7. The following conditions might be associated with this pattern of ECG.
   a. Inferior wall infarction   True   False
   b. Renal failure   True   False
   c. Rheumatic fever   True   False

8. The patient will probably be asymptomatic.   True   False

9. The patient should have prophylactic antibiotics to protect against subacute bacterial endocarditis.   True   False.

10. There are at least three varieties of second-degree heart block.   True   False

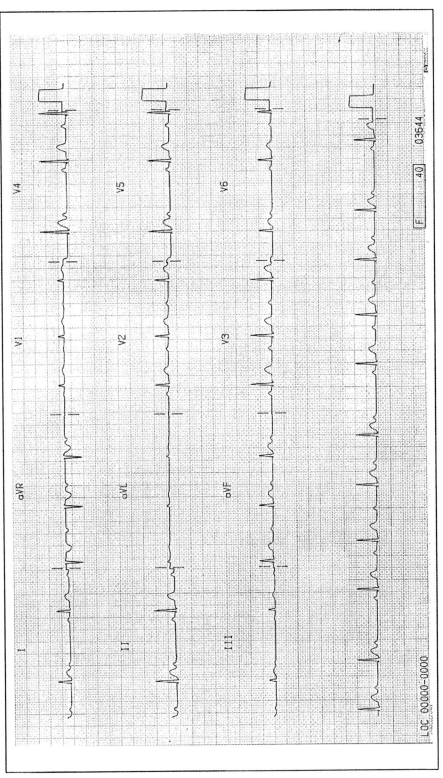

ECG 1

ECG 2

(Answers on page 426)

Questions

1. The vertical deflection on this ECG is less than 1 cm/mV.   True   False

2. This patient should receive antibiotic prophylaxis before any surgery.   True   False

3. There is evidence of spontaneous ventricular activity.   True   False

4. If pacing fails, isoprenaline will increase the heart rate.   True   False

5. Bipolar diathermy is safe for hip surgery in this patient.   True   False

6. The patient would be expected to tolerate a spinal anaesthetic well for inguinal hernia repair.   True   False

7. An MRI scan could be performed safely in this patient.   True   False

8. There is evidence of left ventricular hypertrophy.   True   False

9. There is a right bundle branch block.   True   False

10. Indications for the insertion of a pacemaker include:
    a. Atrial fibrillation.   True   False
    b. Sino atrial node disease.   True   False
    c. Congenital heart block.   True   False

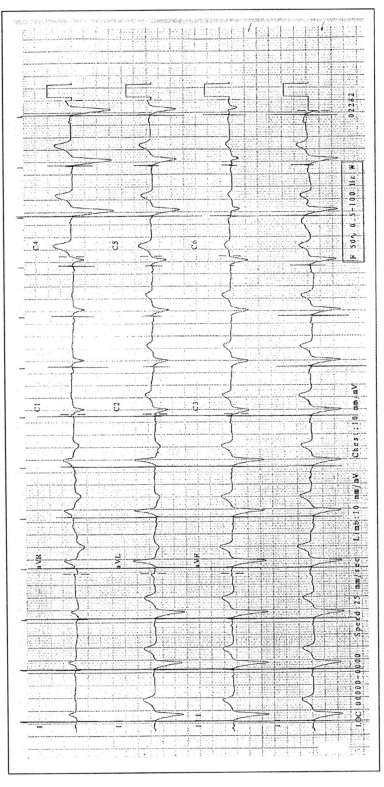

ECG 2

ECG 3

(Answers on page 427)

Questions

1. The speed of the paper is 1 cm per 0.4 seconds. True False

2. There is atrial flutter. True False

3. There is left axis deviation. True False

4. The patient has had a myocardial infarction. True False

5. There is a paroxysmal atrial tachycardia. True False

6. The patient should be given digoxin. True False

7. There is a LBBB. True False

8. It is likely that the patient is breathless. True False

9. There is pericarditis. True False

10. The heart condition diagnosed with this ECG pattern may be complicated by a ventricular septal defect. True False

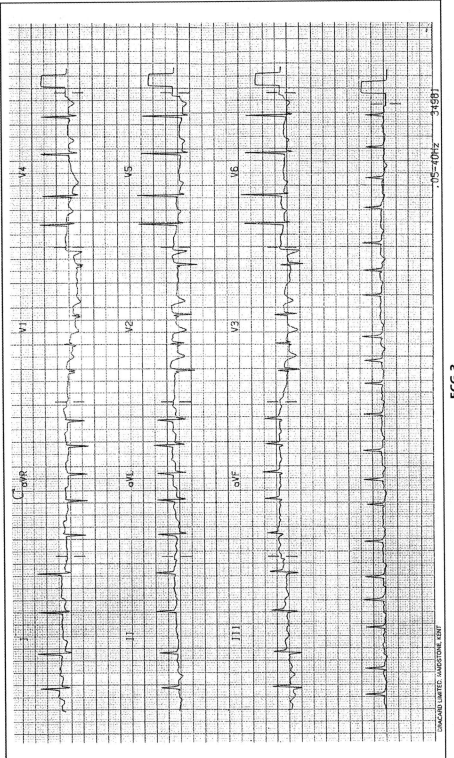

ECG 3

ECG 4

(Answers on page 428)

Questions

1. The heart rate is about 60 beats per minute.   True   False

2. A normal PR interval is less than 0.2 seconds.   True   False

3. There is evidence of left ventricular hypertrophy.   True   False

4. There is evidence of left ventricular strain.   True   False

5. Left ventricular hypertrophy occurs in about half of the patients with mitral incompetence.   True   False

6. There is ECG evidence of left atrial enlargement.   True   False

7. There is ECG evidence of right ventricular hypertrophy.   True   False

8. The ECG changes are compatible with a serum potassium of 2.4 mmol/l.   True   False

9. The ECG shows that the patient may suffer from a prolapsing mitral valve.   True   False

10. If present, a prolapsing mitral valve may be associated with an ASD or a cardiomyopathy.   True   False

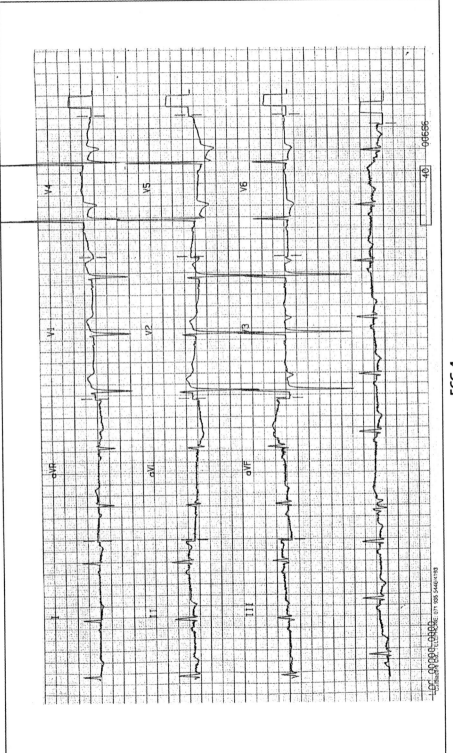

ECG 4

Answers
Electrocardiogram

Answers – ECG 1

1. **False** – The speed is 25 mm/s on the calibration of 0.2 seconds for 5 mm.

2. **True** – Normal axis: the tallest R is in lead II.
Left axis: the tallest R is in lead I with a deeper S in lead III.
Right axis: the tallest R is in lead III.

3. **False** – No evidence of ischaemia.

4. **True** – Mobitz 1 or Wenckebach phenomenon. Progressive PR interval prolongation until one P wave fails to conduct. The QRS complexes are not regular so it is not a third-degree block.

5. **False** – There is no prolonged QRS over 0.12 seconds.

6. **False** – Unlikely as T waves are not tall.

7. a. **True.**
   b. **False.**
   c. **True.**

8. **True.**

9. **False** – No indication for antibiotics.

10. **True** – Mobitz 1, Mobitz 11, two P waves to each QRS. (2:1 block but other patterns may be seen, e.g. 3:1 block).

Answers – ECG 2

1. **False** – The calibration is given by the vertical deflection of 1 cm at the end of the trace.

2. **False** – There is no indication for prophylactic antibiotics in patients with a pacemaker.

3. **False** – All the QRS complexes are preceded by a paced impulse.

4. **True** – Isoprenaline should be available to stimulate cardiac activity if the device fails.

5. **True** – Bipolar diathermy is preferred to unipolar.

6. **False** – The patient has a fixed cardiac output and may develop hypotension if a sympathetic block leads to vasodilatation.

7. **False** – The MRI scanner can interfere with pacer function.

8. **False.**

9. **False** – Right bundle branch block is diagnosed from a QRS complex over 0.12 seconds and an M-shaped complex in the right chest leads. The QRS is about 0.12 seconds due to the spread of the paced impulse in the ventricles.

10. *a.* **False.**
    b. **True.**
    c. **True.**

Answers – ECG 3

1. True – The calibration records a distance of 0.5 cm (5 mm) for 0.2 seconds.

2. False – Atrial fibrillation. Atrial fibrillation is associated with dilation of the left atrium as in mitral valve disease, ischaemic and hypertensive heart disease and thyrotoxicosis.

3. False – The axis is normal.

4. True – ST elevation in V1–3 and T wave inversion in all chest leads. Q waves in 111, aVF.

5. False – PAT is a regular rhythm with T waves fused with the P waves.

6. True – The patient has a fast atrial fibrillation and digoxin would be one treatment, particularly if associated with ventricular failure.

7. False – LBBB is a prolonged QRS of over 0.12 seconds and an M-shaped wave in the left chest leads V5 and V6.

8. True – The patient has had a recent myocardial infarction which may be associated with left ventricular failure.

9. False – Pericarditis is diagnosed by an elevated ST segment through all the chest leads. In this case the elevation is only present in V1, V2 and V3.

10. True – The extensive antero-septal myocardial infarction was complicated by a VSD in this patient.

Answers – ECG 4

1. **True** – The distance between R waves is about 25 mm.

2. **True.**

3. **True** – The deepest S in V2 and the tallest R in V5 add up to over 40 mm.

4. **True** – There is ST segment depression with T wave inversion in V4, V5 and V6.

5. **True.**

6. **True** – The P wave is M-shaped.

7. **False** – Right ventricular hypertrophy will be suggested by right axis deviation and tall R waves in the chest leads with S waves in the left chest leads.

8. **True** – The ST segments are depressed and there are U waves in V2, V3, V4.

9. **True** – There are inverted T waves in the inferior leads 11, 111, and AVF.

10. **True** – It can be associated with both these conditions, as well as Marfan's syndrome, thyrotoxicosis, rheumatic and ischaemic heart disease.

DATA INTERPRETATION 14

Introduction

Each station involving data interpretation is laid out with an artefact or set of results. The artefact may be an ECG or CXR and the set of results from such tests as: haematology, biochemistry, lung function and cardiac catheter studies. First study the essential information that is given. There will be an answer sheet on which you mark your answers, similar to an MCQ sheet but with more questions. All questions will be answerable as Yes/No or True/False.

Data 1

(Answers on page 443)

A patient presents with the following haematological results (normal values in brackets):

Haemoglobin 10 g/dl	(11.5–16.5)
PCV 0.3	(0.4–0.55)
RBC $3 \times 10^{12}/l$	(4.5–6.0)
Reticulocytes 0.3% of RBC	(0–2%)
Platelets $90 \times 10^9/l$	(150–400)
WBC $5.6 \times 10^9/l$	(4–11)

Questions

1. The red cells might show anisocytosis. True   False

2. The patient has a MCV of 100 fl. True   False

3. The patient has a MCH of 28 pg. True   False

4. This anaemia is seen in pregnant patients. True   False

5. The serum B12 and folate should be measured. True   False

6. The patient might complain of a sore tongue. True   False

7. The administration of nitrous oxide for 6 hours causes changes to cells in the bone marrow. True   False

8. Ferrous sulphate could be given to treat this patient. True   False

9. If the patient is blood group AB they could safely receive a transfusion of SAGM blood group A. True   False

10. Blood transfusion reduces the incidence of rejection of some organs. True   False

Data 2

(Answers on page 444)

A 67-year-old patient has had several episodes of paroxysmal nocturnal dyspnoea. The cardiac catheter studies show the following pressures (mmHg):

	Phasic	**Mean**
Right atrium	–	12
Right ventricle	60/5	–
Pulmonary artery	60/30	40
Pulmonary artery wedge	–	27
Left atrium	40/20	
Left ventricle	120/0	–
LVEDP	0	
Aorta	120/60	

Questions

1. The right atrial pressure is normal. — True False

2. The pulmonary valve is stenosed. — True False

3. Pulmonary oedema is likely to be present. — True False

4. There will be a diastolic murmur. — True False

5. There is likely to be a systolic murmur. — True False

6. The mitral valve normally has an area of 7 cm². — True False

7. The patient has aortic valve disease. — True False

8. This condition is most commonly seen in females with a history of rheumatic fever. — True False

9. Echocardiography can be used to assess left ventricular hypertrophy. — True False

10. In this patient the difference in pressure between the left ventricle and left atrium is proportional to the degree of disease. — True False

Data 3

(Answers on page 445)

A 75-year-old woman receiving an oral hypoglycaemic and diet to control her diabetes is admitted following 24 hours of nausea and vomiting with abdominal pain suggestive of appendicitis. Normal values are given in brackets.

Sodium 140 mmol/l	(136–149)
Potassium 5 mmol/l	(3.8–5.2)
Bicarbonate 8 mmol/l	(24–30)
Chloride 98 mmol/l	(100–107)
PaO_2 13 kPa on air	(12–15)
$PaCO_2$ 2.4 kPa	(4.5–6.1)
pH 7.1	(7.4)
Glucose 30 mmol/l	(3.0–5.3)
Urea 15 mmol/l	(2.5–6.6)

Questions

1. The patient has a respiratory acidosis. True False

2. There is an anion gap of 39 mmol/l. True False

3. The normal anion gap is less than 18 mmol/l. True False

4. The patient's condition is compatible with a non-ketotic hyper-osmolar state. True False

5. The ECG will show small P waves. True False

6. A urine osmolarity of 200 mosmol/l is only found with pre-renal failure. True False

7. Initial treatment should include calcium. True False

8. Glucose and insulin would be a safe combination to administer to this patient. True False

9. Dehydration alone could account for this urea concentration. True False

10. The calculated serum osmolarity is 355 mosmol/l. True False

Data 4

(Answers on page 446)

A 62-year-old man complains of breathlessness. Lung function tests show:

FVC 2.4 l (predicted 2.4 to 3.6)
FEV₁ 1.4 l
RV 2.8 l (predicted 1.6 to 2.3)
FRC 3.4 l (predicted 2.2 to 3.3)
TLC 5.9 l (predicted 3.9 to 5.6)
TLCO 4.5 mmol/min/kPa (predicted 5.8 to 8.7)
KCO 0.8 mmol/min/kPa/l

The vitalograph and spirometer trace are shown on page 434.

Questions

1. FEV₁ is the volume of gas breathed out in a normal breath.	True	False
2. The results are compatible with obstructive lung disease.	True	False
3. The TLC can be measured using a vitalograph.	True	False
4. The tests are compatible with emphysema.	True	False
5. Steroids might benefit this patient.	True	False
6. Propranolol may improve this lung function.	True	False
7. This picture can be caused by ankylosing spondylitis.	True	False
8. The ECG may show tall P waves.	True	False
9. The vitalograph trace represents the figures in the data.	True	False
10. The spirometer trace is correctly labelled.	True	False

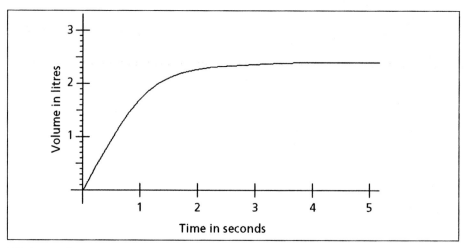

Vitalograph

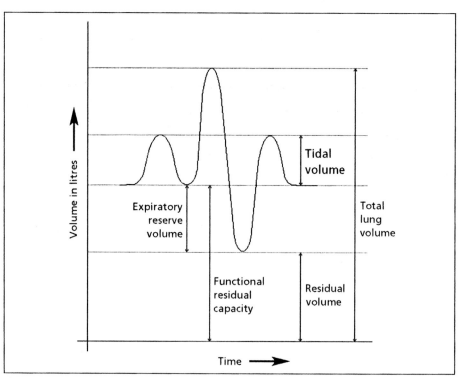

Spirometer trace

A patient is breathless before routine surgery. Pulse and blood pressure are normal. Arterial blood gases show (normal values are given in brackets):

pH 7.55
PaO$_2$ 8 kPa breathing air
Arterial blood saturation 90%
PaCO$_2$ 3.5 kPa
Bicarbonate 20 mmol/l   (24–30)
BEB -4   (0)
Hb 15 g/dl   (11.5–16.5)

Questions

1. The patient will be centrally cyanosed at rest.   True   False

2. The patient will benefit from oxygen by face mask.   True   False

3. The results are suggestive of a metabolic keto-acidosis.   True   False

4. This is an acute situation.   True   False

5. A possible diagnosis would be pulmonary emboli.   True   False

6. The patient will benefit from doxapram therapy.   True   False

7. If the patient is a cigarette smoker the pulse oximeter will under-read the oxygen saturation.   True   False

8. Correcting the alkalosis will lower the oxygen saturation at the same PaO$_2$.   True   False

9. The arterial oxygen content is about 18 ml/100 ml.   True   False

10. The patient should be limited to low concentrations of inspired oxygen.   True   False

Data 6

(Answers on page 448)

The following results are from a preoperative patient (normal values are given in brackets).

Bilirubin 186 µmol/l	(3–18)
Aspartate transaminase 120 i.u./l	(5–30)
Albumin 35 g/l	(35–50)
Calcium (total) 2.14 mmol/l	(2.25–2.6)
Alkaline phosphatase 600 i.u./l	(17–100)
Gamma-glutamyl transpeptidase 25 i.u./l	(10–55)

Urine positive for conjugated bilirubin.

Questions

1. The patient would appear clinically jaundiced.   True   False

2. These findings are typical of alcoholic liver disease.   True   False

3. These findings could be due to gall stones.   True   False

4. These findings are typical of a patient with hepatitis A.   True   False

5. The absence of pain suggests the presence of a carcinoma.   True   False

6. In a preoperative coagulation screen the partial thromboplastin time (PTT) would be a sensitive measurement of the degree of liver impairment.   True   False

7. The serum albumin will indicate whether there is chronically impaired liver function.   True   False

8. Correction of any coagulopathy in this patient should be with cryoprecipitate.   True   False

9. 10 mg of vitamin K should be administered daily until 3 days after the operation.   True   False

10. The prevention of peri-operative renal failure in such a patient should include the administration of mannitol or frusemide.   True   False

(Answers on page 449)

Data 7

Pulmonary catheter pressures

Questions

1. Label the site of the pulmonary artery flotation catheter at each position A to D on the diagram below.

2. The right ventricular pressure is abnormal.　　　　True　False

3. Pulmonary oedema can be present with a normal pulmonary wedge pressure.　　　　True　False

4. The average value for oxygen delivery to the tissues in a healthy adult at rest is 1500 ml/min.　　　　True　False

5. The average oxygen consumption for an adult at rest is 250 ml/min.　　　　True　False

6. Increasing the FiO_2 from 20% to 100% in a healthy person will increase the delivery of oxygen by 25%.　　　　True　False

7. Systemic vascular resistance can be calculated by using the equation: (mean arterial pressure – central venous pressure) × 80 divided by cardiac output
SVP = (MAP – CVP) × 80/CO.　　　　True　False

8. The systemic vascular resistance is reduced by sepsis.　　True　False

9. Pulmonary vascular resistance is reduced by hypoxia.　　True　False

10. Pulmonary vascular resistance is high in cor pulmonale.　　True　False

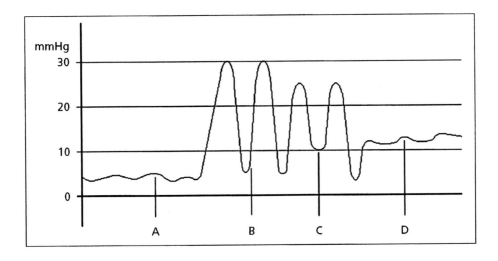

Data 8

(Answers on page 450)

A 23-year-old student is brought to the A & E department by his friend. His friend returned home to find him behaving strangely in his bedsitting room. He has no previous medical history and is physically well.

The following results are available.

pH	7.2
PaO_2	9 kPa
$PaCO_2$	4.8 kPa
HCO_3	18 mEq/l
F_iO_2	40%
Hb	15 g/dl
Pulse oximeter reading	90%

Oximeter reading shows oxygen content of 15ml/100 ml

Questions

1. What does pH stand for?

2. What is the acid base disturbance?

3. What other abnormality is apparent?

4. What is the likely explanation for this man's condition?

5. Why is there a difference in the saturation between the pulse oximeter reading and the saturation from the oximeter reading.

6. If the lactic acid level was 6 mmol/l what condition should be suspected?

7. What treatment should be considered?

Data 9
(Answers on page 451)

A 53-year-old man with long history of peptic ulcer is admitted with abdominal pain and vomiting.

Blood results show:

pH	7.6
PaO$_2$	14 kPa
PaCO$_2$	5.0 kPa
HCO$_3$	28 mEq/l
F$_i$O$_2$	21%
Hb	15 g/dl
Na	128 mEq/l
K	3.0 mEq/l
Cl	75 mEq/l
HCO$_3$	36 mmol/l
BE	>20
Urea	72 mmol/l
Creatinine	90 umol/l

Questions
1. What is the acid base disturbance?

2. How has this change come about?

3. What compensatory changes occur?

4. What treatment is indicated?

5. What precautions should be taken in preparing for a laparotomy?

Data 10

(Answers on page 452)

The following readings have been obtained from a patient

Heart rate	125 per minute
Arterial blood pressure	90/45 (mean 60) mmHg
Central venous pressure	20 mmHg
Pulmonary capillary wedge pressure	10 mmHg
Cardiac output	8.0 l/min

Questions

1. What invasive monitoring device is required to obtain these results?

2. How is the systemic vascular resistance calculated and what are the units?

3. Is the SVR high, normal or low in this patient?

4. What patterns of shock could be present in this patient?

5. What measures should be taken to restore the circulation toward normal?

6. What is the normal adult stroke volume at rest?

7. What is this patient's stoke volume?

8. What would be the most likely cause of pulmonary oedema in this patient?

Data 11

(Answers on page 453)

A pregnant woman has suffered a large APH and following caesarean section has the following blood results:

Hb	9 g/dl
PCV	25%
Red cells	$3 \times 10^{12}/l$
White cells	$3 \times 10^9/l$
Platelets	$70 \times 10^9/l$
APTT	65 seconds
Thrombin time	30 seconds over the control
Fibrinogen	0.6 g/l
Fibrin degradation products	< 1 mg/l
Na	145 mmol/l
K	5.9 mmol/l

Questions

1. What is the likely reason(s) for this picture?

2. What are the main defects?

3. What should be done?

4. What are the possible problems of blood transfusion?

Answers
Data Interpretation

Answers – Data 1

1. True – Anisocytosis is a variation in red cell size often seen with anaemia.

2. True – The MCV (mean corpuscular volume) is PCV/RBC (in this case 0.3/3). Under 76 fl (fl = femto or 10^{-15}) – microcytic cells, over 95 fl – macrocytic cells.

3. False – MCH is Hb/RBC, here 10/3 = 33 pg (normal 27–32 pg, p = picogram pico = 10^{-12})

4. True – Macrocytosis may be due to:
- Deficiency of folate, e.g. diet, pregnancy, cell breakdown as in leukaemia, drugs like anti-convulsants.
- B_{12} deficiency, e.g. pernicious anaemia and lack of intrinsic factor, following gastrectomy, blind loop syndrome, ileal disease, tape worm.
- Other reasons, e.g. liver disease and alcoholism, myxoedema and following heamorrhage associated with a raised reticulocyte count.

5. True – The patient has a macrocytic anaemia – MCV 100 fl.

6. True – Patients with pernicious anaemia have sore tongues, dyspepsia, neurological disorders, liver enlargement and retinal haemorrhages and may have gastric carcinoma. There is an association with certain autoimmune conditions like myasthenia gravis and thyrotoxicosis.

7. True – Nitrous oxide exposure causes inhibition of methionine synthetase activity which will lead in time to megaloblastic changes.

8. False – This is not an iron deficiency anaemia.

9. True – AB is a rare group (3% population), with A and B antigen on the red cells but no serum antibodies. Group A is common (45% population) with A antigen on the red cells and antibodies to B in the serum. These antibodies are washed away in the formation of SAGM blood.

10. True – The incidence of kidney rejection is reduced. The recurrence of some cancer cells may be increased.

Answers – Data 2

1. **False** – Normal 0-7mmHg.

2. **False** – No pressure gradient from the right ventricle to the pulmonary artery.

3. **True** – A wedge pressure above 15mmHg may be associated with pulmonary oedema.

4. **True** – There is mitral stenosis. The PAWP is about the same as the left atrial pressure and at the end of diastole PAWP is higher than LV diastolic pressure.

5. **True** – There are two reasons why this patient is likely to have a systolic murmur:
   - Mitral stenosis due to rheumatic heart disease is likely to be associated with mitral incompetance with the high left atrial pressure.
   - The high pulmonary arterial pressure suggests the development of pulmonary hypertension which will lead to right ventricular failure, dilatation and tricuspid incompetance.

6. **False** – Normally 5 cm².

7. **False** – The pressures and gradient across the aortic valve are normal.

8. **True** – Mitral stenosis is commonest in women following rheumatic fever.

9. **True** – Echocardiography would indicate the size or diameter of the left ventricle. At the end of diastole, a diameter of over 55 mm would mean that myocardial function is likely to remain impaired even after valve replacement. Another indicator of impaired left ventricular function is end diastolic pressure. A pressure greater than 20 mmHg suggests severe impairment to left ventricular function.

10. **True** – The gradient is proportional to the degree of the stenosis.

Answers – Data 3

1. **False** – Metabolic acidosis: low pH, low CO_2 as a compensatory respiratory alkalosis.

2. **True** – The anion gap is the total of all the positive ions (cations) minus the total of all the negative ions (anions).

3. **True** – The anion gap is the difference between the cations and the anions and should be less than 17 mmol/l. An anion gap approaching 40 implies a severe metabolic acidosis, e.g. severe ketoacidosis.

4. **False** – Non-ketotic hyper-osmolar states have a lower anion gap but a higher osmolarity of over 360 mosmol/l. The biguanide oral hypoglycaemic, metformin, can induce a lactic acidosis in patients if taken in overdose, or in the presence of hepatic or renal failure.

5. **False** – The ECG with hypokalaemia shows ST depression, T wave flattening or inversion, prominent U waves which may combine with the P wave to enlarge it. Hyperkalaemia gives small P waves and tall peaked T waves. The QRS will widen and the patient is at risk from ventricular fibrillation.

6. **False** – A urine osmolarity of 200 mosmol/l implies the inability to concentrate within the kidney. It also occurs with the passing of very dilute urine as in diabetes insipidus.

7. **False** – There is no point in giving calcium.

8. **False** – The serum potassium will fall if potassium is not given with the glucose and insulin.

9. **True** – Urea is raised in dehydration due to reduced elimination. This raised urea is not specific to dehydration. Other causes are renal dysfunction and increased protein absoption, e.g. with a gastrointestinal bleed. To assess the degree of dehydration the serum albumin can be used if liver function is normal. To assesss renal function serum creatinine can be used assuming that muscle breakdown is normal as creatinine depends only on renal elimination.

10. **False** – The calculated osmolarity is given by: $Na + K + Cl + HCO_3 + urea + glucose = 140 + 5 + 98 + 8 + 30 + 15 = total\ 296\ mosmol/l$. A deduction of osmolarity can be made by $2 \times (Na + K) + (urea) + (glucose)$. This assumes that the number of anions equals the number of cations.

Answers – Data 4

1. **False** – The volume breathed out in the first second of a forced expiration.

2. **True** – The tests show a reduced FEV_1 to FVC ratio (normal > 70%). The vitalograph only measures for 4 seconds. When the curve is still rising it may underestimate the FVC.

3. **False** – TLC is measured using helium dilution or whole body plethysmography.

4. **True** – The hyperinflated lung and the reduced carbon monoxide transfer factor are typical of emphysema.

5. **True** – The patient might also benefit from oxygen, and a bronchodilator such as a β2 adrenoreceptor agonist (salbutalmol or terbutaline) or an anti-muscarinic (ipatropium).

6. **False** – Beta blockers are contraindicated as they may aggravate bronchospasm.

7. **False** – Ankylosing spondylitis is associated with restrictive lung disease. This pattern of obstructive airways disease can be caused by chronic smoking, living in an environment polluted with dust, cadmium poisoning, α1-antitrypsin deficiency (homozygous), MacLeod's syndrome, Bullous disease of lung, Kartagener's syndrome.

8. **True** – As a sign of right artrial enlargement. P pulmonale results from right atrial enlargement which occurs secondary to pulmonary hypertension from hypoxic pulmonary vasoconstriction.

9. **True.**

10. **False** – The residual volume and expiratory reserve volume have been swapped around.

Answers – Data 5

1. False – Central cyanosis will normally occur when the PaO_2 is < 6 kPa. Central cyanosis requires 5 g/dl of reduced haemoglobin. Peripheral cyanosis depends on local perfusion.

2. True – The patient has a reduced arterial carbon dioxide tension and so does not depend on hypoxia to drive respiration. Oxygen therapy will raise the arterial oxygen tension and saturation.

3. False – A respiratory alkalosis is present.

4. False – The results are suggestive of a chronic, compensated respiratory alkalosis with a low carbon dioxide and a compensatory reduced bicarbonate ion.

5. True – The patient has a reduced oxygen saturation breathing air. This could be due to a ventilation to perfusion mismatch. Possible causes are: pulmonary emboli, lung infection and consolidation, pulmonary oedema. A right to left cardiac shunt could also cause this hypoxia.

6. False – The respiratory drive is intact.

7. False – Carboxyhaemoglobin will be present, half of which will be read as oxyhaemoglobin, giving an over-reading of true oxyhaemoglobin.

8. True – The oxygen dissociation curve is shifted to the right by increasing acidosis or reducing alkalosis.

9. True – Oxygen content = Hb g/dl $\times$ saturation $\times$ 1.34 ml/g = 18.09 ml/100 ml.

10. False – Patients with type I respiratory failure (pink puffers), such as this patient, have a low or normal $PaCO_2$ and do not depend on their hypoxic drive for respiration. Those patients with type II respiratory failure (blue bloaters) have a high $PaCO_2$ and depend on a hypoxic drive to maintain respiration.

Answers – Data 6

1. True – The bilirubin is over 40 μmol/l.

2. False – Gamma-glutamyl transpeptidase is low. The MCV may also be increased in alcoholic liver disease.

3. True – Alkaline phosphatase is raised. This indicates biliary obstruction. The causes of obstruction are gall stones, drugs, e.g. contraceptives, carcinoma of the pancreas and primary biliary cirrhosis.

4. False – AST too low. The AST would be very high in any acute hepatitis.

5. True – No pain suggests carcinoma of the pancreas. Pain suggests cholecystitis, biliary duct obstruction due to gall stones or a distended liver capsule.

6. False – Prothrombin time (PT) is better as it relies on the liver produced clotting factors 2, 7, 9, 10.

7. True – As the liver is the sole source of albumin production a low albumin would suggest chronic liver impairment.

8. False – Vitamin K or fresh frozen plasma should be considered.

9. True.

10. True – The risk of peri-operative renal failure will be reduced by good hydration, mannitol, frusemide and dopamine.

Answers – Data 7

1. **A** – CVP or right atrium
   B – Right ventricle
   C – Pulmonary artery
   D – Catheter in wedge position.

2. **False** – The right ventriclar pressure is normally within the range of 15–25/0–8 mmHg.

3. **True** – If the alveolar endothelim is damaged or if the serum osmotic pressure is low.

4. **False** – Cardiac output is 5000 ml/min and oxygen content 20 ml/100 ml.

   The average value for oxygen delivery to the tissues in a healthy adult at rest is 1000 ml/min. The true delivery of oxygen to the tissues at rest is given by the equation:

   Oxygen delivery = cardiac output × ((arterial oxygen saturation × haemoglobin concentration × 1.34) + (partial pressure of arterial oxygen × 0.023)) divided by 100

   or

   DO_2 ml/min = CO ml/min × ((SaO_2/100 × Hb g/dl × 1.39) + (PaO_2 kPa × 0.023))/100.

5. **True.**

6. **False** – Most of the oxygen is carried by the haemoglobin. The only increase will be in dissolved oxygen at the rate of 0.023ml/100ml blood/kPa.

7. **True** – Calculated as 1000–2000 dynes sec/cm^5. 80 is a correction factor.

8. **True** – SVR is reduced by vasodilators, volatile anaesthetic agents, regional anaesthesia, and anaphylatic, septic and neurogenic shock.

9. **False** – Pulmonary vascular resistance is reduced by nitric oxide and prostacyclin. It is increased by hypoxia and acidosis.

10. **True** – Hypoxic pulmonary vasoconstriction occurs secondary to chronic lung disease leading to cor pulmonale. It is also high in VSD with Eisenmenger's syndrome which can occur in Down's syndrome patients. Its importance is the possibility of a worsening in the reverse shunt with IPPV.

Answers – Data 8

1. The small p means negative logarithm to the base 10. H stands for hydrogen ion concentration.

2. A metabolic acidosis.

3. A low oxygen saturation but a lower oxygen content.

4. Carbon monoxide poisoning from a faulty gas fire.

5. Some of the carboxy haemaglobin will be measured as oxyhaemaglobin by the pulse oximeter.

6. A fire involving cyanide released from burning foam.

7. High inspired oxygen concentration. If the patient is pregnant or severely hypoxic a hyperbaric oxygen chamber might be considered, depending on how accessible it is.

Answers – Data 9

1. A metabolic alkalosis. High pH, high bicarbonate.

2. The man has been vomiting hydrochloric acid and chloride ions from the stomach due to a pyloric stenosis. This leads to a metabolic alkalosis and hypochloraemia.

3. The kidney tries to retain hydrogen ions and loses sodium and potassium. Bicarbonate ions are retained to replace the chloride ions. Potassium is lost as well as sodium. Fluid is lost as vomit. The stomach secretes several litres into its lumen each day.

4. Fluid replacement. The patient requires rehydration with an isotonic fluid. In practice this will be achieved with isotonic 0.9% saline to which potassium chloride has been added. 5% dextrose to which potassium has been added will be used when the sodium concentration is restored to normal and particularly in children to prevent hypoglycaemia.

5. The patient should be rehydrated and the electrolyte balance corrected. This is not an emergency operation. A nasogastric tube should be used to empty the stomach. A rapid sequence induction of anaesthesia should be used, particularly if solid material is still in the stomach.

Answers – Data 10

1. Flow-directed pulmonary artery flotation catheter (Swan Ganz is less precise).

2. Resistance = pressure/cardiac output.

   Systemic vascular resistance = mean arterial pressure – right atrial pressure/ cardiac output.

   80–0/5 = 10–15 mmHg/l/min.

   Convert to cgs units ($\times$ 80).

   This patient has a value of about 400 dyne/seconds/cm^{-5}.

3. Low. Normal is 770–1500 dynes/s/cm^5.

4. Septic, systemic inflammatory response and anaphylactic.

5. Fluids, preferably colloids. Vasoconstrictor.

6. 70 ml.

7. Stroke volume = cardiac output/heart rate = 8000/125 = 64 ml.

8. Acute respiratory distress syndrome (this is not cardiogenic and the PCWP is not raised).

Answers – Data 11

1. Large blood loss and fluid replacement.

2. The Hb is low. This may have been low due to the pregnancy, which dilutes the Hb, but it has fallen due to blood loss and then risen due to blood transfusion. The clotting tests are all prolonged with weakness in the intrinsic system and fibrinogen is not converted to fibrin. The low clotting factors are due to blood loss, dilution of factors and a failure to transfuse and replace enough factors. The platelets are not below the critical $50 \times 10^9/l$ but are low. The fibrin degradation products are low and a DIC is unlikely.

3. A Hb of 9 g/dl does not indicate the need for a blood transfusion particularly as the PCV is low and there may be dilution with isotonic fluids. If there is fluid over load the Hb will rise when a diuresis occurs.

FFP and platelets should be given to improve the clotting and also the albumin level. It is likely that if SAGM blood and isotonic fluids have been given the osmotic pressure will also be low.

If the patient is showing signs of pulmonary oedema or fluid over load a diuretic should be considered. Monitoring of BR, CVP and urine output will be necessary.

4.
- Mismatch.
- Over-transfusion and heart failure.
- Infection of virus, particularly hepatitis, vCJD and HIV, bacteria and parasites like malaria.
- Hyperkalaemia from ruptured cell (not usually a problem).
- Hypocalcaemia and acidosis from the citrate which binds with calcium to prevent clotting.
- Various reactions – urticaria, pyrexia due to white cell antibodies – reduced by filtering, ARDS seen infrequently due to filtering and use of SAGM blood.
- SAGM blood provides only red cells in a high PVC and so does not provide protein and clotting factors.
- Suppression of immunity which may lead to increased cancer spread and increased infection risk.
- Low magnesium, cold, acidotic, high potassium and low calcium may affect myocardial contractility.

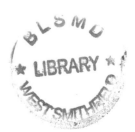